BEING
A
SURGEON
THE TEN COMMANDMENTS

ASAD J. RAJA

MBBS (Karachi), MHSc Bioethics (Toronto), FRCS (Edinburgh)

Quaid-e-Azam Professor and Chairman, Department of
Surgery, Aga Khan University and Hospital, Nairobi, Kenya
and Former Quaid-e-Azam Professor and Chairman, Department
of Surgery, Aga Khan University and Hospital, Karachi, Pakistan

Order this book online at www.trafford.com
or email orders@trafford.com

Most Trafford titles are also available at major online book retailers.

Print information available on the last page.

ISBN: 978-1-4907-8184-6 (sc)
ISBN: 978-1-4907-8186-0 (hc)
ISBN: 978-1-4907-8185-3 (e)

Library of Congress Control Number: 2017905325

Trafford rev.   05/08/2017

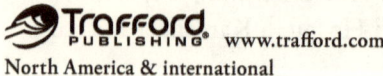 www.trafford.com

North America & international
toll-free: 1 888 232 4444 (USA & Canada)
fax: 812 355 4082

To my dear wife, Rehana, as recognition of her love, unwavering support, and dedication I have received all my life. She has been a true friend, a soul mate, an astute advisor, a staunch critic, and an ardent supporter of everything I do in my life. She knows very well that without her, I am a sail without wind.

To my children, Omair and Zahra, for being true friends, critics, and a joy of my life.

Contents

Foreword

Dr. Raja has taken on a challenging task. How do we convey to the next generation the importance of ethics, morality, and professionalism in the practice of surgery? How much more difficult might that be in the developing world? Dr. Raja is uniquely qualified to attempt such a task. His sense of purpose, moral compass, and ethics shine through in this book. No one will doubt his genuine empathy and desire to ensure that future generations of surgeons do not lose what our generation has worked so hard to cultivate. Some of the stories in this book are strongly colored by the premise of "When in doubt, do what is right." That is a maxim that has certainly guided Dr. Raja.

Some may believe that the battle has already been lost. I, like Dr. Raja, do not believe that. The young people whom I meet as fellows and trainees are as capable, if not more so, than we were. They entered surgery with the same desire to make a difference, as have medical students for generations. They are as intelligent, or more so, than any previous generation; they have absorbed the remarkable expansion of knowledge and understanding of physiology and pathology and have embraced the age of molecular medicine.

Like Dr. Raja, I am concerned that some are retreating from the art of surgical care to be mesmerized by the purely technical aspects of surgical procedures. Minimal-access surgery has brought considerable progress in limiting morbidity. But if we begin to make technology king and the surgeon only a face hidden behind the robot, we run the risk of losing the essential empathy the patient seeks. Dr. Raja is appropriately concerned that as diversity of patient care mandates subspecialization, we risk losing the opportunity to guide and comprehensively manage individual patients. Dr. Raja laments the loss of surgeons as captains of the ship. The opportunity has not been lost; it is there for the surgeon to assume—if not as captain, then as pilot or navigator.

It seems to me that the present generation are searching for that moral compass that initially led them to be physicians. Dr. Raja feels that we have lost much of what defines the complete physician. Some will see some of the comments as simplistic and unobtainable, but no one will doubt the emotional investment and commitment of Dr. Raja in writing this text. All will feel the conflict and angst as Dr. Raja challenges us to accept progress but not to lose our essential professional belief in the value of caring for the entire patient and his or her family.

Professor Sir Murray Brennan, GNZM, MD
Vice President for International Programs
Benno C. Schmidt Chair in Clinical Oncology
Chairman Emeritus, Department of Surgery
Memorial Sloan Kettering Cancer Center
New York, NY
December 2, 2016

Preface

"You talk when you cease to be at peace with your thoughts," said Khalil Gibran. It's tough, living in an atmosphere of silence with an unspeakable moral burden; therefore, I have spoken my heart and mind. This book is for the patients whose doctors have lost professionalism, for the young surgeons looking forward to long and satisfying professional lives, and for the future role of ethics in a rapidly changing canvas of the discipline of surgery.

Medicine has been practiced for centuries under the Hippocratic oath and under the moral values imparted by role models. Hence, it is not surprising to frequently face questions about the value and wisdom of bioethics education. Some ask whether morals and values can ever be taught at this age. Some even ask whether such an education could ever bring about a change in practice. Jean Piaget (1896–1980), a renowned Swiss philosopher and psychologist, deemed moral development an important component of human development. He argued that cognitive or intellectual development controls every other aspect of human development: *emotional*, *social*, and *moral*. Piaget believed that moral development is part of increasing cognitive sophistication.[1] The objective of bioethics education is therefore to bring increasing cognitive sophistication to moral development.

---

1   Saul McLeod, "Piaget's Theory of Moral Development," Simply Psychology, last modified 2015, www.simplypsychology.org/piaget-moral.html.

Medicine has become increasingly complex, and ethical issues have gone beyond the realms of dress and demeanor. The discipline called *surgery* raises many dilemmas and predicaments in everyday practice. In the absence of role models, bioethics cannot be left to tacit understanding and wild interpretation of a few subliminal messages in clinical practice. There is no dearth of hard science, facts, and evidence for our trainees; these are easy, deliverable, and measurable. However, there is little effort to impart the soft sciences, which bring morals and values to debates surrounding patient care.

Bioethics as an academic discipline is a recent development in many countries. Therefore, it is not surprising that *surgery*, which raises many ethical issues and concerns, has very little published discourse on today's issues. This vacuum represents an ideal opportunity to expand the field of surgical education and scholarship. A distinctive bioethics teaching agenda is under development, which will be more of a cultural change than merely an academic exercise.[2]

After qualifying as a doctor, I underwent postgraduate surgical training in the United Kingdom for eight years. Since then, I have lived, worked, and taught in developing countries. The context of my practice is general surgery in resource-poor settings. However, the perspectives I present are applicable to all surgical specialties and diverse settings. Global morals and ethics are no different, but cultural context plays a significant role in the moral decision-making process. This moral diversity must be acknowledged. With increasing globalization, some perspectives from developing countries will help enrich the discourse.

Being a Surgeon is mainly addressed to surgical trainees, young surgeons, and surgical faculty. However, other stakeholders will also appreciate and relate to this moral discourse on the practices and culture of surgery. This is not meant to be a theoretical textbook on bioethics dealing with philosophical theories, principles, and approaches. It singularly focuses on the surgical discipline. It attempts to unpack,

---

2   Asad Jamil Raja and Daniel Wikler, "Developing Bioethics in Developing Countries," *Journal of Health Population and Nutrition* 19, no. 1 (March 2001): 4–5.

analyze, and appreciate the need to integrate the soft sciences and unwritten practices into the discipline. The Ten Commandments are based on cardinal, ethical, and surgical dictums and famous quotations. I have frequently used these in my teachings over the years. The narrative is based on key reflections on morality in medicine. It is an anecdotal account of real cases and personal experiences with overt and covert messages. The stories are powerful and meant to provoke soul-searching and reflection. Surgeons are a breed of their own, living and breathing a vibrant and strong culture. This book attempts to capture the essence of that surgical culture.

I hope that this small effort will help surgeons around the world make a difference in the care of surgical patients, in serving trainees and training programs, and in improving the culture and practices of surgery. There is enough food for thought here for everybody and about everything. This attempt will hopefully bring about a pragmatic approach to and critical reflection on contemporary professional issues and practices. The bottom-line message is to appreciate that although it is essential to provide competent care, it is equally important to ensure that this is achieved in a professional, dignified, and caring way—the true holistic approach to care.

Acknowledgments

I wish to acknowledge and appreciate the critique, encouragement, and support received on the early conceptual version of the manuscript from Drs. Rehana Raja, Jeffery Rees, Asif Hasan, Peter Singer, and Omair Raja, and Ms. Zahra Raja.

I would also wish to acknowledge and recognize all patients, fellows, residents, students, and colleagues who, over the years, have been the great impetus for me to document my thoughts and teachings.

The Ten Commandments

One

WISDOM BEGINS IN WONDER

~

Wisdom begins in wonder.

—SOCRATES

Reflections on the Past

Over thirty-seven years ago, I started my career as a surgical intern in a large teaching hospital in sub-Saharan Africa. There was a perennial shortage of doctors. I was the only intern in one of the surgical firms, and I worked with two trainee surgical registrars and four consultants. I soon realized that I was the workhorse of the department, and I made the unit my permanent abode.

In my first few weeks, I admitted and clerked an elderly African lady with a long-standing, largely asymptomatic multinodular goiter who was planned for a thyroidectomy. She had been rendered almost blind (navigational vision) due to smallpox, which had been contracted when she was a teenager. While obtaining her consent for the operation, I reassured her that this was a routine operation performed every day, that she would be fine, and that she would be discharged in a couple of days.

She was a pleasant and calm lady with a weather-beaten and aged face. She came from a remote village, and despite her blindness, every wrinkle on her face testified that she had seen and endured things beyond my imagination.

She assured me by patting my hand. "Daktari, you sound more worried than me," she said. "I trust you, and you know what you are doing." Being blind and illiterate, she put her thumb impression where I wanted. I was touched and moved by her personality and her trust. Never had I imagined that her words would haunt me forever and shape my career for life.

The next morning in the operating room, I hesitantly tried to discuss my examination findings of retrosternal extension with the consultant. Radiology then was synonymous with plain X-rays and some contrast studies. He looked at the thoracic-inlet X-ray and said, "It will be all right." I dared not ask if he meant that it was or wasn't extending into the chest. Such was the hierarchy and intimidation.

The surgery proceeded, and we found a huge goiter with retrosternal extension. No sweat. The consultant surgeon put his index finger on the side of the gland and into the chest. After some struggle and awkward maneuvers, out popped the large retrosternal component. My eyes popped out, too, as the hole in the patient's chest welled up with blood. Suddenly, I felt I was standing on shifting sand. I was scared for my patient and the possibility of an adverse outcome, which I had never considered. Her words echoing in my ears were interrupted by a shout. "Suck and concentrate!" I then saw a large gauze being tightly packed into the hole. We finished the operation and removed the gauze. To my relief, it seemed dry except for some mild oozing. A drain was left, and the wound was closed.

It was the last case on the list. The consultant left, and I stayed with the patient as she was wheeled to the recovery area. I sat on the counter in the recovery bay and started writing operative notes. I was deeply engrossed in documentation when I slowly started to hear some patient snoring in the background. As the snoring became louder, it occurred to me that it was my patient having a stridor. I rushed to her and found that she was barely arousable and had a large and tense neck swelling. It was already lunchtime, and only a skeleton staff was around. My nurse had left me to fetch some drugs. I had read about a post-thyroidectomy hemorrhage, but I had never seen it.

There was no one around to guide me. The traditional and standard kidney dish packed with the necessary instruments for the emergency removal of Michel clips and the evacuation of a thyroid hematoma was lying at the patient's bedside. I shouted for my nurse, and in the meantime, I gathered the courage to open the wound and evacuate the hematoma. I did it promptly with my shaking hands and lot of prayers. Now I was faced with active bleeding, and I started to panic. I did what I had seen in the operating room: I packed the wound with sterile gauze and asked the nurse to hold pressure on it while I went to look for help. In the changing room, I found our anesthetist. He rushed over, intubated the patient, and asked me to get my surgeons.

The consultant was out of contact on the road somewhere, and there were no cellular phones. Our trainee registrar came in, and we wheeled the patient back into the operating room. We explored, but by then, the bleeding had stopped. We ligated a few small vessels here and there, but we couldn't see well enough to identify what was bleeding in the patient's chest cavity. We left two large bore drains and closed the wound. Now I was permanently stationed in the recovery area. I ran between the patient and the phone, trying to cross-match and get more blood and begging someone to cover my urgent ward work. Two hours later, the patient was still pouring blood, and I sat beside her, pumping blood and watching it come out of the drains.

We finally got hold of the consultant, who came in and decided to pack the cavity, leaving orders to just continue giving blood. By two in the morning, the pack was dripping blood. When we informed the consultant, he told us to call the cardiothoracic team to split the sternum and have a look. We reexplored and split the sternum and found a buttonhole in the right innominate vein. It would stop bleeding in previous explorations due to the extended neck position of the thyroidectomy. We repaired the hole, but by this time, she had received multiple transfusions, developed coagulopathy, and was oozing from everywhere. There were no blood products; if you were lucky, you might get one or two units of fresh blood during the day. Otherwise, it was nothing but stored blood and calcium gluconate. We finished the procedure and removed the drapes.

Just as I was beginning to hope that the patient would live, she went into cardiac arrest. While I was doing a cardiac massage, it seemed that I was the only one who had any conviction in what we were doing. Despite the intubation and despite all the monitors, the drugs, the anesthetist, and the surgeons, the patient could not be revived. At one point, I was told to stop the cardiopulmonary resuscitation (CPR). With much reluctance, my cardiac massage became slow and less forceful, and I don't know when it stopped. She died at six in the morning.

Less than twenty-four hours before, this outcome had not even been in my wildest dreams. I was shell-shocked. I kept staring at the patient; she looked younger because her wrinkles were smoothed out due to puffiness. Her lips were pale, and she had a smile on her face. I stood by her like a guilty child—head down, standing still and speechless, waiting for punishment. I held her hand, and with tears in my eyes, I said, "I'm sorry for not knowing enough, sorry for not doing better, sorry for betraying the trust that I was not worthy of, sorry for letting you down so terribly."

Everybody slowly left, and I was assigned to do the paperwork and perform the last hospital rites with the nurses—all this when I felt mortally wounded, both physically and emotionally. It was nearly twenty-four hours since I had left the operating rooms. I changed and walked listlessly to my unit, where I bumped into the internship coordinator. He told me that since the previous day, I had, to my credit, eight serious-incident reports for not being found to cover my duties in different areas of the hospital. This was typical in a large teaching hospital where the right hand doesn't know what the left is doing. I walked past him almost in disdain. I was lost in the bigger question: What does it mean to be a surgeon or a doctor?

I was not worried at all about my physical endurance, but I was concerned about my shattered dreams and the assault on my values. I had never prepared for such a professional life. Every day, I was being left to obtain patient consent for procedures I knew little about. I had to answer every query from worried patients and families without understanding much myself. I was supposed to alleviate suffering, yet I was inflicting more pain by informing patients that they had cancer or that they needed amputation or that their loved one was being abandoned as a futile case. I was fighting death and certifying the dead. It was a nightmare.

In the early days of my career in the United Kingdom, we received a nineteen-year-old girl. She was a pillion passenger on a motorbike en route to her university in the morning when an oncoming car hit her. She had a bad degloving injury to her right groin—which exposed and damaged her external iliac and femoral vessels—and an associated hip fracture. I called the vascular surgeons.

It was daytime, so their whole team responded with their consultant. They decided that because it was a dirty and exposed wound, any vascular graft repair would have no cover and would get infected. Therefore, they suggested a hip-disarticulating amputation of the leg. I was the first-year resident (SHO or senior house officer) on this orthopedic unit, and she was my patient. I felt the decision was insane, and I could not resist speaking. I politely asked, "Is there any harm in trying? Amputation will always be an option. This way, we are just condemning a nineteen-year-old to a disabled life without even giving her a chance."

The senior surgeons were visibly red. There was a hush of silence and obvious disdain; my comments were perceived as emotional and irrational. The consultant turned around and stared at me over the crowd. After a mortifying pause, he looked over his half-rimmed spectacles and asked, "How long have you been a doctor?" I told him it had been less than eighteen months. He said, "No wonder." I showed no remorse and said no more. They left me standing by the patient as I thought, *Surely, this is not what it means to be a surgeon.*

Later, my own consultant told me that I was reported to him for challenging their decision and being disrespectful. He patted my back and said that he was happy I had questioned their decision. I told him that I was still disturbed with the decision and that it was not about scoring points. I genuinely felt that we should have tried even if there was only half a chance. I thought they should come and see the poor girl's pain now. She was devastated, totally withdrawn, and always in tears. Why was it so hard to think from the perspective of a nineteen-year-old? I thought that being a surgeon was all about trying and fighting; some, we may win, and some, we may lose, but not for want of trying.

The reality was sinking in that caring for human lives and dealing with human beings was not going to be easy. As I was grappling with these new realities, another incident occurred that rocked me to the core. I was halfway through my first six-month training rotation in the United Kingdom in accident and emergency (A&E). One Sunday morning, there were only two of us covering the usually quiet morning shift. This was often a period of lull after the overnight storm of Saturday night. We were alerted by ambulance control that they were bringing in a child who had been in a road-traffic accident. The nurse in charge (sister) and another nurse started organizing the resuscitation room to receive a pediatric trauma patient.

I heard the ambulance sirens and approached the resuscitation room. I saw a stable-looking five- to six-year-old child sitting on the stretcher trolley and being wheeled into the room. A third person walked in with two members of the ambulance crew. He was the child's father. The sister asked him and the crew to make room for the doctor to come in. They turned around and saw me coming toward the room. The father immediately shouted across the room, "I don't want any colored doctor to touch my child!"

I was stunned and froze in my stride. I couldn't decide to go in or to go out. I took a deep breath, composed myself, slowly approached the father, and reassured him that I would send my colleague to see the child. Even before I finished, the sister immediately told the father, "The child will be seen by this doctor and nobody else."

I told her that we should sort out the child and respect the wishes of the father and that I had absolutely no issues with that. "But I have issues. The child is fine, and I am not tolerating any of this nonsense," she angrily snapped.

My colleague, who was listening to the commotion, rushed in and simply refused to see the child. I did not even notice until I heard his voice from behind me, saying, "It's this doctor or nobody, and before he sees your child now, you must apologize to him. You have shamed us all by your racial slur against our very decent and highly competent colleague." I still remember his red face full of anger. There was now an apparent standoff with the father.

By then, I was shaking but overwhelmed by the outpouring of support and solidarity from my colleagues. I was the team leader of the shift, and by now, I could barely speak. But I managed to tell my colleague, "Please see the child; there is no cause worthy of compromising patient care. I am sorry that I am not in a position anymore to see the child."

I walked out to the office. I had put on a brave face. But I was very young and inexperienced, and I felt very low and dishonored. It was the first time in my life I had experienced such a thing. I realized how it felt being considered a lesser human being due to the color of my skin. As I sat there—many thoughts running through my mind and struggling to get my composure back—there was a knock on the door. The father walked in, followed by the sister. He said that his son was all right, and he had come to apologize for his behavior. He explained that he was just stressed out and sincerely regretted his remarks. I thanked him wholeheartedly and explained how important his apology was to me. I reassured him that I had no hard feelings and escorted him back to see his son.

Reflecting back on the early years of my career, I wonder why I was faced with such an impasse. It is difficult to pinpoint one particular reason. However, you could certainly place a sizable portion of the blame on the type of training that we received. There was every emphasis on teaching and evaluating clinical knowledge and skills, but there was little emphasis on human interactions and conflict. Even after entering practical life, there were few resources to help one's moral distress and emotional suffering. This was compounded by the fact that there was neither time to stop and reflect nor anybody to provide counsel. I felt I was made to act like a zombie, and all my compassion, altruism, empathy, and dreams of being a healer were being systematically beaten out of me.

Advocacy

Today, the inadequacies of surgical education and moral development are being exposed. The surgical profession exposes you at a very young and tender age to the day-to-day heartrending realities of human suffering, pain, sickness, and death. The bioethics education you receive these days prepares you to solve some complex ethical dilemmas. But it does not address the everyday moral conflicts that surround caring for one's patients, making difficult and morally disturbing choices, making observations of differential care, practicing surgery under the cover of anesthesia or behind drapes, and living with conflicts of interest. As trainees, living with all these challenges and moral distresses is not easy, but we must never become indifferent. We must always take the moral high ground and make prudent choices, all while keeping our souls as sensitive and human as ever.

Surgical culture is still very hierarchical and parochial in many places around the world. Superiors tend to reign supreme, and there are always attempts to suppress moral indignation. This is inherently unethical. Even if you are right, there must be a humble respect toward others' perspectives. The only thing certain about surgery is uncertainty. We must acknowledge these uncertainties and our own fallible positions.

Trainers must understand the potential to harness the enthusiasm, compassion, and moral instincts of their trainees. First, you must be conscious of the ever-present moral conflicts in the sensitive minds of trainees. You must always be able to read the invisible writing in every wrinkle on their foreheads that reads, "Fragile—handle with care." Never trivialize or stifle them, even if their issues sound insignificant. There are no foolish questions but many intolerant answers. Create a culture of support. They must feel confident enough to externalize their moral conflicts, self-doubts, disillusionments, and despair. Encourage them to open up, ideally by describing your own moral conflicts to receive their advice and opinions. There is nothing more reassuring than exposing your own vulnerabilities as a human being. Harness the inherent desire of the trainees to help the suffering, and go beyond.

The environment you need to foster is not meant to harden and cultivate indifference but to keep trainees soft, enthusiastic, and sensitive. They are looking for that help and support in making the transition to being virtuous surgeons.

Challenges

Surgery is one of the oldest crafts, but it has only been accepted as a scientific discipline for a little over a century. Despite surgery's short history of acceptance as a science, a revolution is in progress. Improved diagnostics and minimally invasive interventions are accomplishing things unimaginable in the recent past. These rapid advancements have changed the philosophy and face of surgery, even during my single professional life. Surgery has become patient centered, with reduced trauma, reduced pain and suffering, improved outcomes, shorter hospital stays, and rapid return to normal life. Surgical diseases have changed their pattern and spectrum; with our better understanding at the cellular, molecular, and genetic levels, the remedies are less and less invasive. Current-day therapies and technologies have already deposited many operations and many surgical dictums into the history museums. And we are nowhere near the end.

It is exciting to be part of this revolution. However, progress and technological advances always bring more issues to light. This is a challenging time on many accounts, especially for trainers, trainees, and young surgeons.

Historically, surgery and medicine in general have been fraught with the trials and tribulations of integrating science and ethics. A surgeon is an eagle who flies with two wings: science and ethics. You must understand that both these wings need to be equally developed and nurtured if this eagle is to fly smoothly, high, long, and far. Currently, the bioethical discourse, tough ethical challenges, and morally disturbing issues are being avoided or abdicated to a battery of dwindling role models. More often than not, you are not aware of what you may be implicitly teaching and what kind of passive learning may be going on in clinical practice.[3] It is important to appreciate that trainees learn more from your practice than from your lectures. Serious introspection is required to analyze and understand how best to develop professional behavior and ethical practices among trainees.

Trainers and trainees must also appreciate that it is our professional and societal obligation to train surgeons and produce good patient outcomes. This is a precarious balancing act, and it is incumbent on us to have structured training programs that rationally and ethically fulfill this dual responsibility.[4] Patients are skeptical about the engagement of trainees at different levels of care. Almost all have no issues with trainees engaging in history taking, physical examination, and general provision of care as a team. However, most patients express reservations about trainees operating on them if they are asked about this unambiguously. Certainly, more patients agree to be operated on by trainees when one reassures them by explaining the concepts of responsibility commensurate with competency, supervision, and consultant responsibility and accountability for ensuring patient safety and good outcomes. Society is still far from appreciating that grooming without mentorship and perfection without practice are impossible.

Programs must be conscious of the supervisory needs of trainees in competency-based training. Trainees must appreciate their responsibility and work within their competencies and limitations. The path to the development of certain skills cannot be abbreviated, so there is no need to compromise patient safety. Just aim to get your foundations strong for the basic and routine surgical work of your specialty. In the prevailing and ever-changing scene of surgery, with all the steep learning curves of new technology, learning should and will continue for one's professional lifetime. Institutions and departments must develop preceptor programs

---

3   Wade Gofton and Glenn Regehr, "What We Don't Know We Are Teaching: Unveiling the Hidden Curriculum," *Clinical Orthopedics and Related Research* 449 (2006): 20–27.

4   Asad Jamil Raja and Alex Levin, "Challenges of Teaching Surgery: Ethical Framework," *World Journal of Surgery* 27, no. 8 (August 2003): 948–951.

for young surgeons after residency. It is important to have such training before you are declared competent for independent privileges and for performing all-new and high-end procedures. Education is for life, and you must be a lifelong learner to progress and achieve success as a surgeon. If the foundations are strong, the sky is the limit; be patient.

Surgical discipline has historically had a strong culture, but the rapidly changing scene of surgical practice is eroding many of the values in the culture of surgery. Culture is an identity and a way of life for any discipline, organization, or society. If it is lost, everything is lost. Despite the huge challenges due to surgery's current state of flux, the core values of surgical culture will never change. The acknowledgment of this fundamental premise is essential for all trainees.

In surgery and ethics, there is therefore a union of science and compassion. Trainees must endeavor to integrate these two elements into the practice of surgery. The training programs and trainees who fail in this effort are likely to suffer a marginalized fate in this journey. All endeavors must therefore be directed to the acquisition of professional and ethical competency and the integration of these into lifelong practice. This will help ease many of the challenges of the tough professional life ahead.

Two

Education is Not Preparation for Life; Education is Life Itself

~

Education is not preparation for life; education is life itself.

—John Dewey

Professionalism

Medical professionalism is widely understood but difficult to describe in a concise statement that satisfies everyone's requirements. The World Medical Association (WMA) white paper "Professionalism and the Medical Association" describes medical professionalism as having the skills, attitudes, values, and behaviors common to those undertaking the practice of medicine. It includes concepts such as the maintenance of competence for a unique body of knowledge and skill set, personal integrity, altruism, adherence to ethical codes of conduct, accountability, a dedication to self-regulation, and the exercise of discretionary judgment.[5]

"Medical Professionalism in the New Millennium: A Physician Charter" is a great document.[6] It advocates a renewed sense of professionalism with adherence and commitment to the principle of the primacy of patient welfare, such as dedication and commitment to serving the best interests of the patient; the principle of patient autonomy, such as being honest with patients and empowering them to make informed choices; and the principle of social justice, such as the need to promote justice in health care, which includes fair distribution of health-care resources and elimination of inequalities and discrimination.

I believe a medical professional must possess three Cs—*character, competence,* and *compassion.* These three Cs are overarching attributes, which I term the *triangle of medical professionalism.* These attributes cut across every facet of professional behavior, and the triangle encompasses every value of medical professionalism under the three traits: *character* (honesty, integrity, trustworthiness, altruism, and justice), *competence* (knowledgeability, possessing required skill sets, current practices, and safety), and *compassion* (empathy, benevolence, caring, and patient advocacy). Deep reflection on and understanding and internalizing all these values are required if we are to model professional behavior. As Khalil Gibran said, "Only if you drink from the river of silence shall you indeed sing."

Unfortunately, the practices of today are far from the values and expectations of professionalism. Nearly a thousand years ago, Al Asuli—a great physician from Bokhara, Persia—wrote a pharmacopoeia that he divided into two parts: diseases of the rich and diseases of the poor. Today, if Al Asuli were alive, he would witness a world even more polarized than that described in his treatise. Today, management

---

5   Jeff Blackmer, "Professionalism and the Medical Association," World Medical Association, last modified July 2007, http://www.wma.net/en/30publications/35whitepapers/White_Paper.pdf.

6   "Medical Professionalism in the New Millennium: A Physician Charter," *Annals of Internal Medicine* 136 (2002): 243–246.

techniques are divided among the rich and the poor. There are distinct levels of differential care between the private and public sector. Even within the private sector, there are levels of care, and treatments are offered based on affordability.

Today, in some countries, if you cannot afford minimally invasive surgery, you are offered an open, invasive procedure by the same surgeon in the same hospital. Medical oncology has different regimens to suit every pocket. Even radiation oncology has linear-accelerator treatment or cobalt radiation therapy depending on affordability. Therefore, if you are poor, you are more likely to suffer the insult and injury of unnecessary open surgery, greater toxicity, and side effects of cheaper oncological regimens; the collateral damage of substandard radiation therapy; and lower success rates.

If you can afford it, you can influence any health-care decision. There are patients who freely access care for lifestyle cosmetic surgery, and there are patients who cannot access care for life-preserving procedures. How ironic and appalling can it become? It is understandable if something is not available; then one gets whatever is available. However, inability to access something when it is available or to get differential care due to lack of affordability is disturbing and unacceptable. Surely, there is something seriously wrong if somebody is dying of thirst while sitting on the banks of the Nile River. What has happened to this world? Where is the duty of care? Where is the primacy of patient welfare and justice? Where is professionalism?

In the late '90s, I was the chair of the Institutional Review Board (IRB) at our university, and I grappled with the consent forms. It always started with the statement in English that "We are planning to do research on . . ." However, when it was translated into the local language, it read, "We are planning to do a study . . ." In the local language, the literal translation of *research* was *experimentation*, and the researchers would argue that if they used the word *experimentation*, no one would consent. I was very uncomfortable with this fudging of language and at being an accomplice to such deception. However, others considered it a norm, and they believed that without it, there would be no research subjects. The onus was left on the research subjects to understand the word *study*. I wondered whether our primary obligation was to researchers or to research subjects. Where is the respect for the autonomy of patients or research subjects?

There are still many great surgeons among us who constantly exhibit the highest level of professionalism. Unfortunately, there are also some others who dishonor the profession. Years ago, as a trainee, I had a very nice colleague from another developing country. His wife, a primigravida, was expecting. He was planning to travel home to be with her for the delivery. One day, I heard him telling his wife on the phone that if she needed to have an emergency Cesarean section, she should tell the surgeons to do a cosmetic incision (a transverse Pfannenstiel incision) and not an up-and-down incision (vertical).

I asked him, "Why would a surgeon even think of using a vertical incision, and why must you worry her with such a thing? It is a professional matter; let the surgeons take care of it."

I was shocked when he replied, "The surgeons there charge more for what they have marketed as a transverse cosmetic incision, and unless you agree to pay more, you just get a vertical incision." It is too generous to call this unprofessional conduct.

Lack of access, differential care, and conscious decisions leading to substandard care due to non-affordability are a big challenge to professionalism today. It is a moral burden, which is impossible to accept or condone. However, instead of anguishing in despair and living with a feeling of helplessness, we must collectively make every effort to thwart such practices. Even if you can make a little difference, it is enough to keep the fight alive. Otherwise, after a while, we will forget the difference between right and wrong, and we will start accepting atrocities as norms of practice.

I sincerely believe that there is hardly anyone who does not understand and appreciate the values and expectations of professionalism. However, several fall short when it comes to practice. This is due to competing motives, which are at times overwhelming. But we must not forget that we have chosen to be in a profession with some fundamental expectations from the profession and society. We must reflect deeply and challenge our consciences to live up to these societal and professional expectations.

I was once travelling on a domestic flight in South Africa. As the plane was taxiing before takeoff, the usual inflight air-hostess announcement said something unscripted: "If due to any reason, the cabin pressure drops, an oxygen mask will fall in front of you. First, help yourself by tugging and putting the mask on your face before you help the children. Among the children, help would-be doctors first and would-be lawyers last!" There was a burst of laughter on the plane. It was a great ploy to keep people attentive and interested, but there was a subtle message in it, too. The medical profession is still very highly regarded by society. This makes it all the more important for young surgeons and trainees to live up to the expectations of this highly revered profession.

Duty of Care

There is an expected duty of care as a medical practitioner once a patient-doctor relationship is established. This is a direct, formalized contractual relationship, but there are many other complexities to such a relationship that are beyond the scope of this discussion. Understanding the basic premise of this principle and its ramifications is central to the practice of surgery.

In tort law, a duty of care is a legal obligation imposed on an individual requiring adherence to a standard of reasonable care while performing any acts that could foreseeably harm others. It is the first element that must be established to proceed with an action in negligence.[7]

I believe that besides a legal compulsion, a duty of care is also a moral obligation. It is imposed on caregivers and requires adherence to a standard of reasonable care (judged at the level of your peers) while performing any acts that could foreseeably harm the patient. Duty of care also entails the disclosure of risks and alternatives to the patient so that

---

7   "Duty of Care," Wikipedia, https://en.wikipedia.org/wiki/Duty_of_care.

informed choices can be made in order to avoid harm. Harm caused by not fulfilling the duty of care or by acts of omission or deviation from standards of care without any solid grounds may amount to negligence. Daniele Bryden, an anesthetist and health lawyer, states that to establish negligence, one needs to prove the following three things in a court of law: that the doctor owed a duty of care to the patient; that the duty of care was breached; and that as a direct result of this breach, the patient suffered harm.[8]

I will outline three surgical cases concerning how medical negligence can come into play and where an expectation of duty of care may or may not have been breached. I leave it up to the reader to judge whether and where there may or may not have been a case for medical negligence.

A surgical colleague of mine was on call one night, and he inherited a twenty-one-year-old patient who was admitted in a moribund state from a remote village of another province three days after the onset of acute abdominal pain. He was obtunded, very sick, in septic shock, and severely acidotic, and he presented with a board-like abdomen due to peritonitis. While he was being resuscitated, he went into cardiac arrest in the emergency room (ER). CPR was performed, and the patient was revived after eight or nine minutes. A plain abdominal X-ray revealed pneumoperitoneum, and a clinical diagnosis of enteric perforation was made. All this occurred in the ER—in no-man's-land—while the surgeon was sleeping at home. Now with a surgical diagnosis, the patient was admitted under him.

The surgeon came in during the middle of the night and saw the patient for the first time in the intensive care unit (ICU). The patient had already been intubated, was post-CPR, was suffering from septic shock and on inotropes, and had an acute abdomen. Given that he was a young patient with a treatable disease, he was taken to the operating room. The family was spoken to (despite the language barrier) and clearly told about the brain insult he may have suffered and that the general outcome may not be good. During surgery, the cause was found to be an ileal

---

8   Daniele Bryden, "Duty of Care and Medical Negligence," *Continuing Education Anesthesia Critical Care and Pain* 11, no. 4 (2011): 124–127.

perforation, possibly due to typhoid fever. The surgeon exteriorized the perforated terminal ileum as a loop stoma and did a copious washout. The patient did well and recovered except for the hypoxic brain injury that he suffered during CPR. He was now in a persistent vegetative state (a coma-like state where eyes are open with the appearance of wakefulness rather than true awareness).

Hospital personnel explained the situation to the family. But the family blamed the surgeon and the hospital for negligence. According to them, when they brought the patient in, his brain was fine; he only had abdominal complaints, and all the damage occurred after the surgical procedure. Was the duty of care breached here, and were the relatives justified in their claim of negligence? If so, was the surgeon to blame or the ER doctor or neither?

A forty-five-year-old obese patient sustained a single gunshot wound. The entry wound was in the epigastric area, and the exit wound was over the right flank near the iliac crest. A laparotomy revealed two holes along the trajectory, one in the right transverse colon and the other in the ascending colon. The patient underwent an extended right hemicolectomy with primary anastomosis. On day three, he suddenly manifested signs of sepsis and rapidly entered septic shock. He was intubated, resuscitated, and brought to the operating room on inotropes and tapering urine output.

A computerized axial tomography (CAT) scan was not performed due to hemodynamic instability and renal dysfunction. A nonenhanced scan in an immediate postoperative abdomen would not have added much value. Reexploration revealed no intra-abdominal catastrophe, but it did reveal an edematous whole right flank along the long track of the exiting bullet, which had developed severe necrotizing fasciitis. The skin outside looked normal, as is usually the case. This required extensive debridement.

Soon after surgery, while the patient was still on the table, he developed cardiac arrest. CPR was unsuccessful. An arterial blood gas (ABG) test done just at the end of the procedure revealed severe metabolic acidosis with hypercarbia. The end tidal carbon-dioxide levels were very high throughout the surgery, and the patient had no urine output during the procedure. The ventilator machine had a respiratory rate setting of fourteen per minute throughout the procedure. Was the standard of care breached, and did it cause direct harm to the patient?

A fifty-year-old obese female patient underwent major elective pelvic surgery. Postoperatively, everyone assumed she was on prophylactic anticoagulation for deep venous thrombosis (DVT). However, she had only received compression stockings and had been encouraged to perform early ambulation. On day six, she had a massive pulmonary embolism from which she could not be revived. Was there an act of omission or a deviation from the standard of care, and did it result in direct harm to the patient?

Surgeons must be careful with what they conceal and what they reveal. It is understandable at times not to be up-front about rare complications unless the patient poses a question. Even a minor operation can be fatal, but we never talk about it. The intention is purely not to burden the patient with remote risks and unnecessary worries. There is a risk of dying while crossing the road, but we don't warn anybody of that risk because it is so miniscule. However, it is your duty of care to disclose any sizable risks and alternative choices while obtaining consent from a patient.

Unfortunately, doctors have become obsessed with the legal duty of care. They have become paranoid due to litigation-prone environments. The duty of care should always be extended with a spirit of moral obligation. The issue of litigation is important, but it should be a secondary factor. You should never allow it to devolve into a situation of all form and no function, such as seeing the patient for two minutes and documenting for twenty minutes. It is understandable that care not documented is legally considered care not given, but you must at least provide the care required before you start documenting. Defensive practice of medicine defeats the spirit of the duty. It is expensive and a waste of resources, it can be a source of physical and financial harm, and it may still not save you in a court of law. The spirit of duty should be paramount over any other consideration in the provision of care.

Acculturation into the Surgical Discipline

Over the years, I have asked almost every prospective candidate interviewed for the residency program, "Why do you want to do surgery?" The most common answers are the following: surgery is different, it's exciting, it's rewarding and gratifying, and one gets instant results. Some always knew they wanted to do surgery whereas some thought they were more practical and good with their hands, and certainly all had abundant passion for surgery. I can assure you that I have challenged all those statements; I have asked why all may not be true for other specialties. To me, surgery is different from other specialties in countless ways. It is necessary for aspiring and trainee surgeons to grasp this perspective. This will help them understand why we are different and why we must be different. It is important to foster this surgical mind-set early.

Surgery is different from other disciplines because it is inherently invasive. You must first inflict more insult and injury to already-sick people before you can make them better. This surgical decision-making—its timing, extent, and competence—has direct bearing on the outcomes. The knife in the hand of a surgeon can be a double-edged sword. Although it has the potential to do good, it can also be a source of immense harm. Surgery is not all glory, and it is chilling to see how horribly things can go wrong. Most often, the reasons are multifactorial, but bad outcomes can also be due to poor surgical judgment and surgical incompetence. Therefore, it is not surprising that surgery is associated with pain, suffering, complications, repeated procedures, disability, and even death. There is more fear of surgery than of any other specialty in medicine. Surgery is therefore a serious business for the patient, and so it should be for the surgeon.

The high expectations and professional demands of surgery differentiate our mind-set, approach, and attitude from those of other specialists. In emergency settings, surgical patients are particularly vulnerable because of urgency and limited choices. Usually, resident teams on call initially deal with these emergencies during odd hours. The management of these patients in the proverbial golden hour significantly impacts outcomes. These teams must be competent and vigilant. Any delays, inappropriate management, or lack of appreciation for the gravity of the situation can lead to disastrous consequences. Consultants are happy being on call with a resident who has an acute sense of responsibility, is thoughtful, and has a low threshold for raising the alarm. On the other hand, in elective situations, patients are well informed, and they have choices. They wish to scrutinize everything before they may or may not agree to a surgical intervention. We must develop credible structures and systems at all levels of surgery to improve patient trust and confidence in both emergency and elective settings.

Surgery is different from other specialties. Because it is a craft, patients tend to chase established names, gray hair, and a credible reputation. New surgeons face a difficult period trying to get established as surgeons; they sometimes unnecessarily end in difficult situations with adverse outcomes. The advice to them will always remain the same: There is no shortcut to this set-in period. Be patient; tread carefully. Make good choices, and carry them out well. Never yield to any external or internal pressures. The willingness to ask for help is a strength, not a weakness. Keep an unassuming profile, and let your work speak for you. One good thing about surgery is that you cannot hide your outcomes. If you are good, nothing stops you. Chase the highest standards of professionalism, and a great and everlasting professional reputation will chase you.

Surgery is diametrically different from other specialties; we don't deal with outpatients and inpatients only. We spend more than half of our practicing life in the operating rooms. This is our workshop, where we have our team and the tools to apply the craft of surgery. It is a place that tests the character—as well as the physical and mental endurance—of even the best of us. It is a place where one does not see the light of day. In cumulative hours, surgery may take up a sizable part of your lifetime. One must therefore understand this place—its dynamics and its nuances—to ease some of the challenges of this life.

The operating rooms host rendezvous of surgeons, anesthetists, residents, medical students, scrub nurses, technicians, runners, porters, and housekeeping staff. It is a place where you can do a case study on the improvement of team dynamics and win a Nobel Prize. The team at best is an assorted bunch who can be a pleasure to work with. More often than not, one is frustrated to no end—from starting the case to positioning the patient, to adjusting lights, to having someone who knows what one is doing, and to having the right tools that work: a diathermy that sounds and works on the first go, equipment that kick-starts without a fiddle, a sucker that actually sucks and a sucker bottle that is not emptied at the most crucial point, supplies that don't go out of stock during the operation, saline for irrigation that is not too cold or too hot, and a swab and instrument count that is correct the first time around.

This is a worldwide phenomenon, but it is compounded in resource-poor settings. This challenge can be minimized by team development, but it can never be eliminated. If a flowing river is unable to dislodge a boulder from its way, it doesn't stop. It just flows around it and moves on. Don't lose your cool; be aware of such irritants, and learn to work around them or with them. Never curse your setup or tools. We don't live in an ideal world. Surgery is no exception. There is no place for anger or aggression, and if the leader has lost it, then don't expect anything better from anybody else. Always look at the bigger picture. At the end of the day, the patient and the outcome are your responsibility. Remain focused on the patient.

The other most frustrating and time-wasting period is the patient turnaround time (TAT) in the operating rooms. This is one thing that most surgeons get worked up about that makes the operating room atmosphere tense, which is not good for anybody. It can also adversely impact the procedure one is performing. One's true character comes to light in the face of adversity. Show your composure, and rise above everything as a team leader. You must understand the most important principle of your career: It is only in the interest of the surgeon to finish the operating list. The interest of the other team members is just to finish the shift. In other words, the surgeon works by looking at the operating list, and the other team members work by looking at the clock.

How can you ever beat this conflict? Just back off, and cool down. In my experience as a chair of a teaching-hospital department and as the chair of a theater users' committee, I have not been able to make any significant dent in this issue. I am always shown good statistics of improved TATs, but the ground realities are different; forget the statistics.

I also believe that somebody could be writing the twenty-fifth edition of this book, and this issue would still be relevant. Set an example, always be on time, bring the patient to the operating room yourself if necessary, and put in the Foley catheter or the intravenous (IV) line while you wait for the anesthetist. The patient will see that you care, and your fellow staff will realize that if they will not do something on time, you will.

These days, we have smartphones, tablets, and computers with Wi-Fi access everywhere. You can use operating room time in between cases intelligently instead of getting frustrated. Trainees can read about an operation that has just finished or about one that is just about to start. Surgeons can sit and reflect on the procedure, on what worked and what did not, and on how they would do things differently next time. They can plan the procedure about to be performed. No matter how many times you may have done something before, each case is different and requires the same attention, insight, and care. Therefore, utilize your time in the theater productively instead of pacing up and down the operating room corridors like an expectant father. Come prepared not to be irritated by things beyond your control.

Managing a surgical patient on a medical floor can be quite challenging. The needs and requirements of each surgical patient are different, and the medical team is simply not geared toward handling surgical patients. It is like leaving your car with a motorbike mechanic just because he is also a mechanic. You can give the medical team a new elective admission or a convalescing patient who is on his or her way out. But trust me, you should get your patients on the surgical floor under your team. Otherwise, be prepared to suffer a lot of distress and even disasters. Similarly, thinking that it is sufficient to leave patients in semi-open critical-care areas with the four walls, equipment, technology, and staff there is foolish. Own your patient, and never abdicate your responsibility. Critical-care staff is well trained and do their best; however, their performances are individual and variable. They do bring a lot of strengths and expertise to critical care, which is crucial for the team, and you bring your surgical expertise and experience—co-manage the patient. The patient is ultimately your responsibility; it is your name on the patient's headboard.

Surgical discipline is an amazing merger of science and craft, and you can do a lot of good if you are sensible, disciplined, and persistent. There can be nothing more gratifying and rewarding than when a young lady walks into your clinic, happily carrying a newborn baby. She is profoundly grateful to you for saving her and the baby. After the initial embarrassment, you finally remember that about five months ago, you did a splenectomy on her when she was five months pregnant. She was a diagnosed case of idiopathic thrombocytopenic purpura and was on medical treatment for a year. She was admitted under the medics as an emergency with a platelet count of one thousand, severe subconjunctival and petechial hemorrhages, and melanotic stools and at a risk of developing large spontaneous hemorrhage anywhere, anytime.

On the other hand, there can be nothing more depressing and demoralizing than when a fifty-two-year-old dies on the day of discharge after an uneventful right hemicolectomy for carcinoma colon. He had stable myelofibrosis for six years and was living on platelet counts of sixteen thousand to seventeen thousand with no adverse events. On that fateful day, he walks to the ward toilet in the morning, and a Valsalva maneuver results in a massive intracerebral bleed on a platelet count of twenty-eight thousand. What do you tell the family when you are called on the floor to explain? How does one satisfy them as to what went wrong? All your surgical science, evidence, and statistics have failed you and fail to pacify a distraught family.

Surgery has glory and success, but there is also adversity. It can be very unforgiving and cruel. The nature of the discipline requires you to have lot of humility. Always stay grounded; if you become brash, you will soon receive the slap of an adverse outcome. It is important to be kind and gentle to others in morbidity and mortality (M&M) meetings. Always first acknowledge the difficulty and complexity of the situation and the huge advantage of hindsight. These forums are meant for reflection and not for humiliation.

Surgeons are different from the commonly advanced perception that we are mere technicians. We take pride in the definition of a good surgeon as one who is an excellent clinician and a deft technician. It is our fundamental professional obligation as *surgeons* not to act as *technicians* for anybody, ever. One may be invited to an already prepared and diagnosed patient who is ready for surgery. Take ownership of the patient and make up your own mind, diagnosis, and management plan. This is not an ego issue; it's the best practice for the patient, and it demonstrates respect for the discipline of surgery. Acting as second fiddle to someone else is unprofessional and can be of immense harm to the safety of the patient. Bad practices of surgery are detrimental and expensive.

The surgical discipline is losing its surgical craft to technology at the speed of light. Today, there is no orifice in the body—normal or abnormal—that an endoscope has not been developed to enter. Even a small fistula-in-ano can be repaired with an endoscope. Minimally invasive interventions in many areas and specialties are making surgeons superfluous. Then there is robotics; anything you can imagine is either here or in the works. The way things are moving, open surgery may become obsolete in a short time. This is all good for the patient and the future of the profession. Specialists and trainees must keep pace with new technology and continue acquiring new skill sets. We must learn to understand, guide, influence, and manage these transformations. Losing your craft to other people and specialties due to complacency is a recipe for becoming redundant and being sidelined even faster than obsolete technology. This is the time for the surgeon to embrace his or her care of the patient as we embrace new techniques. These are desperate times; protect your turf.

Surgery is different because it disturbs you emotionally as you constantly struggle with life and death. The ones you save keep you going and balance the anguish and pain of the ones you could not save, who can scar you forever.

I had a young colleague, a plastic surgeon, cry on my shoulder. The beautiful baby on whom he did a perfect, uneventful cleft-lip and cleft-palate repair did not wake up from anesthesia. This was all in a tertiary-care center and in collaboration with the most senior and experienced pediatric anesthetist. The whole team was devastated, and the mother was distraught and hysterical. She kept saying to the surgeon, "I gave you my child. You return my child back to me." This is when the stark realism of surgery is overwhelming as a surgeon.

Trauma, tumors, and terrorism inflict the most horrible scars on your mind, especially through children and the young when they die in your hands and you cannot do anything. And when things go wrong in your hands despite your best intentions and efforts, it can prick your conscience forever. Surgeons have the highest number of skeletons in their closets—enough to overwhelm you with eternal humility.

Finally, trainees must appreciate that every culture knows illness, and every culture makes provisions for the ill. There is a lot of suffering, disease, disability, death, and bereavement, especially in surgery. The culture of surgical practice must also ameliorate this suffering; we are doctors before we are surgeons. We must appreciate that in addition to physical suffering, there is mental, emotional, psychological, social, and economic suffering, which unfortunately barely surface on our radars. This suffering often continues long after the physical wounds have healed, even sometimes for life. Loss is part of the journey of life, and it also teaches us what is precious and valuable. The values of humanism served by medicine stem from the journey of our shared experience of illness, love, compassion, and caring. In surgical culture, we must place immense importance on upholding these values of humanism and on fostering enduring human relationships.

Three

Develop a Passion for Learning; You Will Never Cease to Grow

~

Develop a passion for learning; you will never cease to grow.

—Anthony D'Angelo

Self-Discovery

It is ironic that we avidly read and try to understand and analyze everything that comes our way but rarely bother to read and understand ourselves. This journey of self-discovery is at least important when making a choice about specialization in any discipline of surgery. It is essential to appreciate your strengths and weaknesses, likes and dislikes, wants and desires, and many other things. All these are necessary to shape the temperament of an individual. Surgery is one discipline in which temperament plays a major role. Temperament, from the Latin *temperamentum* (proper mixture), is defined as a mixture of your nature, personality, character, disposition, perseverance, temper, outlook, and spirit.[9] I am sure you would like to have the best attributes of all of them. But do you have that temperament? Is it intuitive? Can it be cultivated?

I think all of us have an innate level of the basic ingredients of all these attributes. But how well they have been nurtured is a reflection of one's upbringing. If the broad, basic ingredients are right, there is always an opportunity to impact and improve on the desired attributes, provided that there is enough desire. As you exploit your strengths, it is important to simultaneously work on your weaknesses. If you are unable to surmount your major weaknesses, then you are likely to struggle as a surgeon. Dealing with life and death is not a part-time occupation. If you cannot tolerate the heat, then don't stand near the fire. The burden of self-appraisal and making choices lies with the trainee. Others will only know of your shortcomings when it may be too late. Therefore, these early decisions and choices go a long way in shaping your future career.

Once you have decided to become a surgeon, roll up your sleeves and jump in. In surgery, there is very little room for people with hands in their pockets. Be a true professional. Don't just *go* through your training; *grow* through your training. Developing and growing up as a surgeon has many facets that need a lot of work, dedication, and commitment. Nothing in life comes easily, and surgery is more demanding than any other profession. Indeed, the best surgical expertise is bought at the cost of great pain and sacrifice. Discipline yourself and persevere. There is no such thing as routine in surgery; everything must be well thought out and done with a purpose.

A word for trainers: We must not belittle our role in creating an enriching environment for our trainees to enable them to grow, flourish, and mature. I once planted at my home two trees in the front garden and four trees in the rear garden. All of them were of the same species, age, and height, and they were planted at the same time and in the same manner. A year later, the four in the rear garden were growing tall and blossoming, and the two in the front garden were half their size and really looked miserable and unhappy. A friend visited me and was baffled by what he observed. I told him that this is what a fertile, enabling,

---

9   "Temperament," Dictionary.com, http://www.dictionary.com/browse/temperament.

and nurturing environment will do to anybody. You can select the best of society, but an inappropriate environment can ruin them. Therefore, creating and developing an enabling environment is crucial and should be a hallmark of every good training program.

Reflective Practitioner

Surgery is invasive; it is a source of trauma and insult to already-sick patients. This iatrogenic trauma must be very controlled, timely, and well calculated. This is called *surgical judgment*: knowing when to do something and, more importantly, when not to do something. In surgery, it is said, "A good surgeon knows what to do, and the best surgeon knows when not to do." Good surgical judgment is crucial to obtaining good outcomes. It is a complex phenomenon acquired through experience. There is no substitute for experience, but merely experiencing something does not make you wise or astute. It is the reflection on the experience (good or bad) that ultimately enriches your mind to make judicious decisions in the future.

Critical thinking and reflecting all the time during practice are therefore essential for experiential learning and the development of good surgical judgment. There are three models of *reflective practice* described and practiced in medicine. Donald A. Schön (1983) described the first two models for reflective practitioners.[10] One is *real-time reflection*, when you are going through an experience (reflection *in* action). For example, you are treating a patient in hypovolemic shock; after fluid resuscitation, you feel that the patient is now adequately hydrated, but there is still no urine output. You give a diuretic challenge, and there is still no urine output. Now you wonder whether you are trying to squeeze a dry towel or whether the filtration is clogged. You reflect back again on all the subjective and objective parameters and try to make new assumptions in favor of one or the other possibility. Subsequent decisions will be based on this real-time critical reflection during delivery of care. Real-time reflection is dynamic and requires instant decisions.

---

10   Donald Schön, *The Reflective Practitioner: How Professionals Think in Action* (San Francisco: Jossey-Bass, 1983), 123–135.

The second reflection is *after the event* (reflection *on* action). For example, you have just finished a trauma laparotomy, and you sit down as an individual or as a team and reflect on the experience. What worked, what did not, and why? This critical reflection is crucial for learning because the events are fresh in the mind, and this reflection must happen after every experience, big or small, good or bad. We all know that after every event or experience, there is always room for improvement and learning.

The third model for reflection, described later by Killion and Todnem (1991), is about *reflection for future actions* based on all past experiences (reflection *for* action).[11] This is a reflection on the cumulative experience of M&Ms, case series, audits, practices, and so on, and these then come to bear on our future decisions.

These three types of reflective-learning processes, which happen at different points in time, are crucial to the development of surgical judgment. You can only improve if you constantly reflect on the current and previous experiences and outcomes by continuous self-appraisal. You cannot be repeating the same steps and expecting a different outcome; if you put chicken meat in a mince machine, expect to have chicken mince and not beef mince coming out on the other side. Wise people also learn from other people's experiences and hence enhance their learning experience during reflections at audit meetings. Good surgical judgment is essential to the success of any surgeon, and you must be a reflective practitioner all your life to develop good surgical judgment.

Enquiring Mind

Develop an enquiring mind as a surgeon. Enquiry begins with the search for knowledge and information, and the lack of availability of satisfactory answers is the beginning of research. Then one works on the *how* questions to develop appropriate methodologies.

---

11 Jollen Killion and Guy Todnem, "A Process of Personal Theory Building," *Educational Leadership* 48, no. 6 (1991): 14–17.

There is still a lot of dictum and dogma in surgery that need to be questioned. You may be surprised to find that many well-ingrained practices don't have much evidence to back them up. The majority of procedures have never been put through any scientific inquiry. Most have been refined and modified over the years. They are practiced on the basis of theoretical plausibility and their outcomes. We are still not sure about many new and popular procedures. Many procedures have so many variations and local adaptations that it is astounding to see the differences, even just on the two sides of the Atlantic. And if one looks at the other parts of the world, it sometimes seems that the surgical animal has changed its species and evolved into something else.

On the other hand, there are some parts of the world whose practices and scientific literature are not easily accessible. I am sure they are doing wonderful work, too. Therefore, one can appreciate how incredibly varied and amorphous the practices of surgery are around the world. All are treating the same diseases, albeit sometimes in different manners, and all seem to be faring well and claiming to have good outcomes. Therefore, there is considerable opportunity to learn from each other and conduct research to improve our practices.

We must understand the limitations of surgery and science to subject procedures to randomized, controlled trials. This has been done. But it is difficult and often impossible due to so many confounding variables, and this raises many ethical concerns. Diversity in practice will remain with us, and we must aim to work within accepted norms and principles of practice. Adventurism is unnecessary and may compromise patient safety. As much as one may like and encourage lateral thinking, too much of it is not good; neither is misplaced focus. Young surgeons and trainees must focus and challenge practices with an open and enquiring mind. Any major changes or digressions from the current norms must be monitored carefully and undertaken in the context of prospective data accumulation and, where feasible, clinical trials.

Learning and research are obtunded if you are economical, manipulative, or dismissive of observations and facts that are difficult to comprehend. For example, while taking a patient's history or conducting a physical examination, we sometimes gather information that does not fit in the diagnosis or the developing picture. The common tendency here is to ignore what one doesn't understand. That is the end of learning or meaningful reflection. Never do it. On the contrary, always keep the issue alive. If one continues to think, reflect, and look for explanations, one will always find answers. There is nothing in this world that is without a purpose or a reason. We may not understand it, and then it becomes a question for research. But don't be dismissive of unexplained observations. Enquiry is the best practice for the patient, your own learning, and the advancement of science.

A long time ago, a very fit and healthy forty-year-old business executive was admitted under my care. He presented with a three-day history of a large bowel obstruction. He was a workout fanatic and had nothing in his history to suggest anything leading to this event. The plain X-ray showed dilatation of the right half of the colon up to the splenic flexure, and everything was collapsed distally. A double-contrast barium enema revealed an abrupt cutoff just proximal to the splenic flexure, with no mucosal lesion. There were no colonoscopies or CAT scans in those days. I treated him conservatively. But his condition did not improve, and eventually, I did a laparotomy.

What I found was amazing. All the omentum hanging from the transverse colon had rolled itself into a mass and was adhering to the retroperitoneum in the left upper quadrant in the infracolic compartment; it was like a plugged hole. Distal to this rolled mass, the descending colon was collapsed, and proximally, the colon was massively dilated up to the caecum. The adhesions of the mass of omentum to the retroperitoneum were soft and inflammatory. I just teased them out with my fingers, and everything opened up. The gas reached the sigmoid colon in two seconds. I looked around for any organic pathology in the colon or in the retroperitoneum, but I could not find anything. I closed him up.

I remained baffled about the cause and worried that I might have missed something. I was also annoyed with myself because the patient's condition might have settled with a bit more conservative treatment, and the laparotomy may have been unnecessary. I explained to the patient and his wife almost apologetically that I could not find anything. I had no explanation as to why this had happened and no idea if it would happen again. He had an uneventful recovery and was discharged from my care after the clinic visit for the removal of sutures as he remained well. I could not resist thinking about the cause of this strange case, but I never found an explanation.

One afternoon, about six months later, I was doing my clinic when this same couple walked in. Seeing the patient, I could not believe my eyes. This big, healthy, muscular young man had been reduced to half his size since I had last seen him. I was shocked. Immediately, I thought that I might have missed a malignancy. It turned out that soon after he was discharged from my clinic, he started having low-grade evening fever, which was later accompanied by night sweats, poor appetite, and gradual weight loss. He otherwise remained asymptomatic. He was initially treated by their general practitioner and later sent to an internist, who investigated him extensively for pyrexia of unknown origin. He was then referred to an infectious-disease specialist. The couple decided to consult me first before they went somewhere else.

I immediately knew I would get my answer today. My focus was unexplained disease pathology in the retroperitoneum of the left upper quadrant. I just asked him to hop up on the couch and expose his back. I could just barely see a mass in the suspected area—and only because I knew what I was looking for. I felt a smooth, painless, left paraspinal mass in the lower thoracic spine region over the eleventh- and twelfth-rib area. The clinical diagnosis was obvious: paravertebral tuberculous cold abscess.

I looked at the chest X-ray, which was reported as normal, and it did grossly look normal. However, I focused on the abdomen below the diaphragm, that is, the lower left corner of the film on the eleventh and twelfth ribs in the left lumbar area. I saw a clear soft-tissue shadow suggesting a mass in which both the ribs were completely eroded and destroyed. His erythrocyte sedimentation rate (ESR) was 135. Aspiration revealed typical tuberculous pus, which was positive on Ziehl-Neelsen (ZN) staining for mycobacterium. He was started on antituberculous medications, and he recovered fully after the course of treatment.

On another occasion, I was referred a twenty-eight-year old young woman who had been newly diagnosed with insulin-dependent diabetes and presented with an acute three-day history of deepening jaundice, pale stools, and dark urine. Upon examination, she looked well, and the only finding besides deep jaundice was a palpable epigastric mass. A CAT scan revealed a large, complex cystic mass (ten by nine centimeters) replacing the head of the patient's pancreas. The bile duct was stretched and compressed posteriorly over this heterogeneous cystic mass. The pancreatic duct was massively dilated, and the entire body and tail of the pancreas was completely atrophic. Everything fitted in the picture. The diabetes, atrophic pancreas, dilated pancreatic duct, and the size of the cystic mass all suggested a long process, but why such a short and sudden history of jaundice? No clear explanation came to light at that time. Surgery was planned for about twelve days later.

The patient was readmitted a day before surgery and reported that the jaundice had markedly improved, as well as the color of her stool and urine. Examination revealed that jaundice was considerably reduced and that the mass was now half its previous size, which immediately explained the shortness of the period of jaundice. An acute hemorrhage into this complex cyst (tumor apoplexy) had produced the sudden presentation with jaundice and also brought the tumor to light. We operated, and it confirmed what we expected. Answers are always there as long as you are prepared to keep reflecting on unresolved dilemmas and keep searching for answers.

We must also endeavor not to accept a ready-made diagnosis. Patients come and give one a diagnosis rather than tell one what is wrong with them. This diagnosis is an opinion of another doctor or a referral note or from accompanying investigations. Today, it usually means the patient or his family has consulted Dr. Google. It may all be correct, but your MD is still better than Dr. Google. It always pays to start fresh with an unprejudiced mind. Trust your ability to obtain a good history and physical examination to make a clinical diagnosis, and then confirm your clinical suspicions with laboratory and radiological investigations. It cannot be vice versa with an attitude that all investigations are normal, so let's go and examine the patient now. With such practices, you are likely to miss things and cause unnecessary physical and financial harm to your patient.[12] This will also cause you to gradually lose the ability to make your own clinical judgments. If you listen to the patient long enough, he or she will lead you to the diagnosis.

Similarly, don't read radiological reports before you have reviewed the scans or pictures yourself. First, you will get better at reading them this way, and second, with experience combined with knowledge of the case, you may sometimes pick up things that the radiologists may have missed (like the paraspinal tuberculosis patient above, who had a reportedly normal chest X-ray). These are crucial skills to develop, especially in resource-poor settings.

Recently, I saw a fifty-five-year-old male in my clinic. He was an uncle of a colleague sent to me with a ready-made diagnosis of symptomatic gallstones and ultrasound pictures of cholelithiasis. He was mentally prepared for a laparoscopic cholecystectomy. Despite the fact that he was a colleague referral, I never digressed from the principle of independent investigation. I set aside all the previous investigations and preconceived notions, and I asked the patient to tell me what was wrong with him.

He had a nearly eighteenth-month history of gradually worsening, colicky abdominal pain. The pain was central, starting two to three hours after meals, lasting for a couple of hours, and eventually settling down until the next meal. There was associated heaviness, fullness, and nausea, but he never vomited. He did not notice any alteration in his bowel habits. Previously, these episodes had been infrequent and less severe, but in the last couple of months, they had become regular and severe. He had lost seven kilograms, and he attributed this to poor appetite and being afraid to eat. Despite having lost weight, the patient was still moderately obese, but except for mild anemia, he had no positive examination findings. The giveaway was the classical history, anemia, and weight loss. A clinical diagnosis of subacutely obstructing, right-sided colonic malignancy was made. A colonoscopy confirmed an almost-obstructing

---

12 Sunita Shah, "Investigations Before Examinations: 'This Is How We Practice Medicine Here,'" *JAMA Internal Medicine* 175, no. 3 (March 2015): 342–343.

adenocarcinoma of the ascending colon. He underwent a right hemicolectomy and never had a laparoscopic cholecystectomy.

Another sixty-two-year-old patient recently presented to my clinic with a referral note and a ready-made diagnosis of reducible umbilical hernia for mesh repair. The patient did not mention any problems except for the umbilical swelling. She was entirely focused on it, and she was keen to be operated on. But upon examination, she looked like somebody who had something more serious brewing. Exposure and examination of the abdomen was enough to give away the diagnosis. It revealed fullness of both flanks and a wide-necked umbilical hernia with a positive cough impulse.

The telltale signs were, a two centimeter hard nodule in the umbilicus over the edge of the hernial neck and moderate ascites. I asked the patient if she had lost weight recently, and she described a ten-kilogram weight loss in the last three months. The patient and the family were shocked when I told them the problem was more sinister than an umbilical hernia. An ultrasound, CAT scan, and cancer antigen 125 (CA 125) later confirmed advanced ovarian malignancy. One cannot emphasize enough the importance of an independent enquiry; without it, you are likely to miss things, which could be detrimental for your patient and for your own practice in many ways.

The other skill crucial to the practice of surgery is anticipation. We surgeons are responsible for creating many preventable problems, simply because we never anticipated what was coming. We are often not proactive; we are always reacting and firefighting. There are very few patients who deteriorate suddenly. The majority of patients always give enough warning of deteriorating organ function manifested by subtle signs. Unfortunately, we fail to recognize them or treat the manifestation; we don't step back and look at the whole patient to head off the evolving catastrophe.

The most common example of this in surgery is an evolving sepsis; unfortunately, this is most often diagnosed when the patient crashes with septic shock and multi-organ dysfunction or failure. Many cases of M&M unfortunately results from the following: delays in recognition;

lack of adequate, appropriate, and timely interventions and resuscitations; and lack of appreciation for the gravity of the situation.

It is heartening to see that many good centers have developed rapid-response teams (RRT) to rescue patients manifesting subtle signs of distress. There are modified early warning scores (MEWS) being recorded on wards, and critical scores are immediately communicated to RRT so that they can rush to rescue these patients. However, where we don't have RRTs in hospitals, there is nothing stopping the surgical team from taking the initiative to respond to early warning scores. I call this a preemptive strike, and any team should be able to deliver it whenever it is needed.

There is another dictum peculiar to the practice of surgery: Never do investigations that you would not pursue. The exercise of running a battery of tests every day as a routine is common practice in many places, especially in critical-care areas, where the patients are being co-managed. How does doing C-reactive protein (CRP) and procalcitonin levels every day help or change anything? On the other hand, whenever and wherever there is a possibility of obtaining evidence—such as tissue for a biopsy or fluid for biochemistry or cytology or pus for culture sensitivity— the opportunity is often missed. The bottom line then is "No tissue, no issue" and "No pus, no fuss." Certainly, doctors need to be more sensible and reflect on some of these erroneous practices. Think of the financial resources that could be directed to other needy patients or more important areas if we stopped doing investigations that cannot change patient outcomes.

In emergency and critical-care settings, you should worry about a patient you don't have a diagnosis for. These are the cases in which you are likely to miss something. Serial examinations and frequent reviews at short intervals will elucidate most problems. The patient either gets better or settles down if there is nothing serious brewing, or the patient presents classical features pointing toward a particular pathology. These are classical situations in which reflection *in* action comes into play. Never abandon a patient for whom you don't have a diagnosis or a clear plan. Sometimes, it may be too late by the time you come back. Emergency surgery and surgical critical care are tough and demanding, but they can be enjoyable and very rewarding, too.

Deft Surgical Hand

A surgeon is an artist. The craft of surgery requires a deft surgical hand to execute the operative plan to perfection and fruition. Ease, gentleness, fluidity of movement, dexterity, and experience make a deft surgical hand. There is no substitute for practicing and training with good, skilled surgeons; this is essential for the development of a deft surgical hand. Theoretical knowledge as well as excellent clinical and surgical skills are both equally important.

Surgical skills training should always start in skills labs, in simulated conditions, and on animal material. It is not fair to allow the skills development of novices during live surgery. These days, every skill—open or minimally invasive—can be taught in a simulated and virtual environment. This is true for all specialties and for almost every procedure. Modern and advanced skills labs with simulators and simulated conditions should therefore be an integral part of any major teaching hospital. During and at the end of the training, these skills must be evaluated. Once one has had sufficient practice and achieved competencies in different skill sets, then one can gradually move toward working with real patients.

The best way to achieve real-life skills development is by observing, assisting, and operating with skilled and experienced surgeons. Take it as a privilege to scrub in with masters of the craft, and never miss such opportunity. Develop good observation and anticipatory skills, and understand what is being done. One cannot learn to drive by reading driving manuals; one has to get out and drive with an experienced instructor. This opportunity will not be there once you have finished training. Seize it.

Surgical assistance is an art, and it comes from theoretical knowledge of the procedure being done. Never come to the operating theater without knowing all the patients on the list and having read about all the procedures. You may not be doing the procedure, but this does not mean you should just switch off. You must know exactly what is going on, and it's best to be one step ahead. Anticipate what the surgeon will do next and how you can assist. This is how a good assistant becomes a good surgeon.

Operative-care and skills development starts as soon as the patient enters the operating room. The patient only knows you, and being with your patient when the patient is awake shows that you care. Sometimes, holding the hand of a frightened patient during induction for anesthesia is very reassuring for the patient in an unfamiliar environment where he or she is surrounded by unknown capped and masked staff.

In any kind of surgery, there are several crucial steps before one puts the knife to the patient and before the patient is wheeled out of the operating room. These have direct bearing on the outcomes, and they must be understood and appreciated. You should be wary of the resident who shows up when surgery is about to start and expects to be taken through the procedure as if surgery were all about cutting. Remember, surgery is not a procedure; it's a discipline. Procedure is only a part of the discipline; what happens before (decision-making, timing, and preparation) and after the procedure (care and avoiding and detecting complications) is crucial to the outcome. Engage yourself fully in the patient's journey through the hospital; there is learning at every step.

At M&M meetings, one of the commonly considered causes for an adverse outcome is technical failure. This simply means that the failure of the surgical procedure performed (such as anastomotic leak or wound dehiscence) was due to host factors, surgeon factors, or both. The surgeon factors are due to poor surgical technique or poor execution. Even wound infections can occur due to poor surgical technique as a result of contamination or leaving dead necrotic tissue, hematomas, or tight, strangulating sutures, which produce ischemia. Good surgical skills and tissue handling as well as following the principles of surgical techniques are crucial.

In trauma and emergency situations, the operative field may not look as pristine, calm, or civilized. But in elective, planned surgeries, the operating room atmosphere can give you an idea of the surgical technique and skills of the team leader. It should never look like a battleground. In a controlled, predictable environment of elective surgery, the scene must be the practice of art and craft at its zenith. Minimal blood loss, clean and neat anatomical dissections, use of appropriate instruments rather than hands and fingers, respect for tissues and tissue planes, and display of calmness and control even at the most crucial steps of the procedure are all hallmarks of safe, competent, and skilled surgery. Speed is important but not at the expense of compromising the safety and principles of surgery. This scene of elective surgery should be ingrained in the trainee's mind for life.

The learning does not end with creating the last stitch. The last crucial step is documentation. It helps one crystallize all steps of the procedure and the aftercare. Always obtain feedback from the surgeon, and have your operative notes checked for accuracy. This vital information will stay in the patient's file for life. Imagine people reading your notes five or ten years later; not only would they have any information they required, but they would also have an impression about the author of those notes. This is true for every assessment and documentation you make in a patient's medical records, and documentation is your only defense in a court of law.

There is a famous saying in surgery that by operating with a bad surgeon, one only learns what not to do. You must work with a good surgeon who teaches you how to be a competent, level-headed surgical team leader. This apprenticeship is crucial to the practice and mastery of all aspects of surgery, especially the development of a deft surgical hand.

Four

A LIVING PROBLEM IS BETTER
THAN A DEAD SOLUTION

~

First, Do No Harm

Why does anyone need to be reminded of this principle? You would be surprised how many times one must repeat this in clinical-care areas or in multidisciplinary-team meetings. Still, one gets a distinct feeling that there is doubt in some eyes when you are reiterating it. The tendency is that as soon as you see a plum, you just want to pluck it. Even in life, you make prudent choices and only bite at what you can chew or chip at issues one at a time or pick and choose your battles or even learn and accept to live with some problems. All this cannot be less applicable to surgery. You may decide to do something, prioritize options, stage the procedure, and do only what is necessary and may even decide to do nothing—yes, doing nothing is also an option. What is the big deal about it? The question is not that because you can do it, so you should do it. The question is much bigger: *Should you do it?*

One often comes across situations in which an intervention has resulted in a maximum adverse outcome; and clearly, there was an alternative of not doing anything, which would require living with disease but would have a significant chance of survival.

A seventy-four-year-old was presented as a postoperative mortality. He was a chain-smoker and had hypertension, diabetes, obesity, mild chronic-renal failure (CRF), a sedentary lifestyle, and poor functional class, and he was now diagnosed with non-small-cell lung cancer. The medical and radiation oncologists struggled with their decision about chemoradiation because he was a very high-risk case due to his CRF, his multiple comorbidities, and his poor functional class. The surgeon thought that surgery would be a lesser evil, so he performed a pneumonectomy.

The patient had a stormy postoperative course and died after twenty-five days. The surgeon felt that the patient had no option but surgery, and the risks were explained to the patient. The patient's comorbidities were optimized, and physicians classified the patient as a high-risk case. According to the surgeon, the procedure was technically sound and uneventful; the patient was extubated in the immediate postoperative period. He had no complications from surgery, but unfortunately, he died of his other comorbidities. The surgeon was asked if he believed the patient would still be alive if he had not done the surgery. Had he considered the option of not doing anything?

Most primary gastric lymphomas are high grade in nature, and the primary treatment is chemotherapy with or without radiation and H. pylori eradication therapy. Surgery is rarely indicated except for complications. We once discussed the mortality of a fifty-five-year-old patient. He had a very large high-grade lymphoma of the stomach extending from below the gastroesophageal junction as a proximal gastric cancer and producing an upper gastrointestinal bleed. The surgeon had to go in as an emergency because there was no angio-embolization, and the surgeon decided to do a total gastrectomy.

Postoperatively, the patient developed a leak of the esophagojejunal anastomosis, and after a prolonged stormy course, the patient died.

During the audit meeting, the surgeon was asked why he had not considered a lesser option in such an acute emergency setting (like devascularization), especially when these are very chemo-responsive tumors with good prognoses. He said he felt that removing the bulk of the diseased organ would save the patient from subsequent complications and would result in a better likelihood of cure. This is like ensuring that one dies of the cure rather than dying of the illness.

I was once asked to consult on a patient who had a large wound dehiscence and fecal fistulas. She was a young lady who had presented five weeks previously with an incisional hernia and a large, lax abdominal wall. She was obese with a body mass index (BMI) of thirty-two, and she had chronic obstructive pulmonary disease (COPD). The hernia was uncomplicated, and she underwent an elective mesh repair for incisional hernia and abdominoplasty.

The mesh got badly infected and was removed, and a washout was done. Later, the patient developed a burst abdomen for which she visited the operating room again for washout and closure. It dehisced again. She was taken back for closure, and while her surgeon was separating adhesions, a bowel segment was devascularized for which a resection anastomosis was done, and the wound closed. The anastomosis leaked and formed a fecal fistula with a large dehiscence. While this was being managed as a controlled fistula with dressings, another fistula developed from the exposed loops.

Now the patient had a large dehisced wound with bowel loops exposed and stool pouring out from two holes. This demonstrates that there are times when it is absolutely fatal to jump into such hostile abdomens with edema, friability, and sepsis. You are likely to cause more harm by either devascularizing tissues or making hole(s) in the bowel. When the wound dehisces the second time and there is no evisceration, you can then just let it heal by secondary intention instead of attempting to wash out and close again. This is a significant morbidity involving a prolonged course of dressings and an incisional hernia, but that is still a lesser evil than the above patient's situation.

Sometimes, it is obvious that masterly inactivity is the best course. But it is not easy to make this decision, and you may not be left with other, better options. Sometimes, calculated risks must be taken.

In the early '80s, in my neurosurgery rotation, we had a young man with a vestibular schwannoma with a classic history and presentation. We were then one of the few neurosurgery centers in the United Kingdom with a first-generation single-slice CAT scanner, which then had applicability to the head only. We also had a continuous ultrasonic suction apparatus (CUSA) for the resection of such tumors. The tumor was benign but large, and surgery was the only option. The patient was young and had a very jovial character. He walked into the hospital, and except for the issues of balancing himself, worsening hearing, and tinnitus, he was up and about on the ward. I remember that the patient and his wife were very positive and looking forward to having the surgery and going home.

The next day, our senior neurosurgeon operated, and I assisted him in this five-hour operation. We used a suboccipital retrosigmoid approach because it was a large tumor, and this approach allowed us to get a better exposure and a better view of the brain stem. The aim was complete resection, and we just ended up debulking the tumor because it was close to the brain stem. Every time we used the CUSA in that area, it produced bradycardia, and we had to stop. Eventually, we abandoned the attempt because it was getting very risky as we got closer and because partial removal is also an option for large tumors. Postoperatively, the patient had a sudden cardiac arrest during the night and could not be revived. The family was devastated, and so were we. But did we have a choice? In those days, we would have still done the same thing in a similar patient. Today, with the option of radiation by stereotaxic means and with the current-day understanding, technology, and support, the outcomes would be much better.

There is a common saying: "If it ain't broke, don't fix it." Given that surgery is a craft, there will always be pressures to do something, even if the patient is fine and has no complaints. Never yield to such pressures; hold your ground to avoid harm. Recently, a sixty-year-old patient with chronic renal failure on twice-weekly dialysis and on steroids for rheumatoid arthritis presented to physicians. He had a ten-day history of fever and no other complaints, and he was referred to us for an urgent consult for a perforated duodenal ulcer (DU).

We rushed to see this patient on the high-dependency unit (HDU), only to find him sitting up in bed. He was having his midmorning tea and snack and chatting away with his wife, who was sitting by his bedside. The story was that during a screening for pyrexia of unknown origin (PUO), the chest X-ray revealed air under the right hemidiaphragm. The patient looked fine; he had no abdominal complaints or findings. They ordered a CAT scan of the abdomen with oral and intravenous (IV) contrast. The scan showed a tiny streak of oral-contrast leakage from a sealed perforated DU into the subphrenic abscess, which had a pocket of air in it. Everything else was fine. Except for the fever and some leukocytosis, the abdomen was benign, and the patient was tolerating his diet.

We decided to do no operative intervention. We got a percutaneous ultrasound-guided drain put in the subphrenic abscess, sent the pus for culture, and started him on antibiotics and proton-pump inhibitors. We advised the team to continue his diet and said we would keep an eye on him. The medical team thought we were crazy for treating a perforated DU conservatively. The consultant later called and requested to transfer the patient under my care. I reassured him that the patient had serious medical conditions and would be better off under their care and that we would continue to comanage the patient. There was no indication for surgery because the perforation was old and had almost sealed off.

A week later, we removed his drain when it stopped draining, and there was no further collection revealed on the ultrasound. His fever settled, and so did his leukocytosis. We stopped his antibiotics and left him under medical care after ten days. Remember, treat the patient, not an X-ray or an investigation. Sometimes, masterly inactivity or minimal intervention is required if the patient is well; otherwise, you are likely to cause more harm.

Clinical examination and modern imaging modalities are picking up what are now commonly being called *incidentalomas*. This is a bad choice of name because it denotes a common pathological entity that is clinically inert. This is hardly the case. It should only be called an incidentally found lesion in an asymptomatic patient. Some of these so-called *incidentalomas* are being picked up on CAT scans and magnetic-resonance imaging (MRI), such as adrenal tumors, renal tumors, pituitary tumors, pulmonary nodules, and retroperitoneal tumors; others on abdominal ultrasounds, such as incidental gallstones, uterine fibroids, ovarian or renal cysts; and yet others on carotid duplex ultrasonography, such as thyroid and parathyroid incidental nodules. Many of these incidentally found conditions are serious and require work-up and appropriate interventions. However, there are some that are relatively benign, such as nonfunctioning, small adrenal adenomas; asymptomatic gallstones; small renal cysts; or small, asymptomatic, multinodular goiters that provoke no cosmetic worries. These things should be observed, but they don't necessarily require action.

There are about twenty different types of tumor markers available currently. These are being used to diagnose and evaluate response to treatment, identify recurrence, and guide prognosis. They are wonderful tools in the field of oncology if they are used judiciously and wisely. Unfortunately, they are being searched for too often in many places around the world. This mindless exercise is driving patients crazy; it's even being called *tumor-marker terrorism*.

People are roaming around with abnormal reports, and they are totally asymptomatic. In many cases, a tumor marker is done randomly to screen for God-knows-what, even though most don't have much diagnostic value in terms of sensitivity and specificity. A normal level does not exclude cancer, and an elevated level does not always indicate cancer; it may not be specific to an organ or tumor. Why do something that helps little in anything and causes havoc in everything? It becomes a witch hunt, and no matter how much one reassures the patients, they live in fear that there is something brewing inside. Some even start repeating the test at regular intervals on their own. Then they come back with a report that is a few decimal points up or down, and they want a physician to make sense of it.

Screening asymptomatic but high-risk patients for any disease is a good method for detecting early disease based on the evidence. However, such screening must be specific and focused, not a random shot in the dark. Otherwise, the current casual practices will continue to cause concern and even be a source of physical and financial harm.

Discretion Is the Better Part of Valor

There is very little difference between bravery and recklessness, and there is no place for recklessness in surgery. The price of failure is too high. Everything has to be carefully thought out, calculated, and planned. Unfortunately, despite all this, one often sees that discretion is overwhelmed by instincts of valor, at times with disastrous consequences. Things must be done based on scientific rigor and need and not based on personal whims or any other extraneous influences, such as peer or social pressures.[13]

Some things are difficult for patients to accept. Having a stoma, even a temporary one, is not easily acceptable. But there may be better understanding and acceptance in some places. There are understandable pressures on surgeons, and they stretch their valor to its limits in avoiding a stoma. Some even believe and preach that giving a stoma is a defeatist approach. Leaks are common; and in a high-risk, elderly patient, this spells doom. It does not end there. Unfortunately, some even try their luck the second time when they go back to wash out; they again don't defunction but try to suture over the leak or patch it with omentum. This is catastrophic. Time and again, one witnesses patients with severe sepsis and multiorgan dysfunction leading to significant morbidity and mortality. This is because of unnecessary valor and prideful belief in one's technical prowess, as well as a lack of appreciation for the confounding forces that create a no-win situation.

There is a general expectation that elective surgical patients should be reversed and extubated from anesthesia in a timely and successful

---

13 Chunzi Jenny Jin et al., "Pressures to 'Measure Up' in Surgery: Managing Your Image and Managing Your Patient," *Annals of Surgery* 256, no. 6 (2012): 989–993.

manner. Some anesthetists, admittedly under pressure from surgeons, unfortunately have taken this upon themselves as some kind of yardstick of success. Stretching this practice to emergency situations in very sick patients is a failure to appreciate different physiological needs and responses to the evolving pathological situation. There will be patients after emergency surgery who can be clearly reversed and extubated. Others are equivocal and may need a delayed extubation once they're settled and stable in the critical-care area. Yet others will clearly require ventilatory support until they revive. That period could be anywhere from a few days to a few weeks. All these situations need a rational approach, and a conscious decision should be made after objective evaluation of individual patient conditions; there is no bravery or cowardice here.

Our fellow in surgery once took an elderly patient of mine to the operating room. He was a diabetic, and he had presented with severe necrotizing fasciitis. In such patients, it looks like a very innocuous disease on the surface, but a storm is brewing beneath the skin, which may only display blistering. The patient was already in sepsis, with subtle manifestations of early organ dysfunction. He underwent an extensive debridement, which is always associated with blood loss. After the major insult of surgery, blood loss, and sepsis, the patient was now in septic shock and multiorgan dysfunction. He was on double inotropes and was tachycardic and severely acidotic with marked tachypnea, and he had minimal urine output. Unbelievably, he was deemed fit for reversal from anesthesia and extubation.

As the patient was being shifted to the critical-care unit, he arrested. Why could we not see what was coming? Later in the M&M meetings, they emphasized that the patient was so sick and moribund that it resulted in the adverse outcome. This may be true, but we did not help the situation. There must be better reflection on how we can help such sick patients by anticipating the need for critical organ support.

There are many other examples of unwarranted valor, such as attempts to resect unresectable tumors, especially in dangerous situations (like indolent, low-grade lymphomas). This usually results in complications or reduces you to a situation in which you are cutting and cracking through tumors all in the name of debulking, performing an anastomosis where a stoma is clearly indicated, and attempting a resection where diversion is indicated. Instead of staging the procedure, you are performing it as one stage, combining removal of a benign, incidental finding with the primary surgery, all at times with very unpleasant experiences and outcomes.

There is no suture or technique yet developed to overcome the brutal and unforgiving pathological forces of sepsis, malignancy, and other states. Additionally, failure to appreciate and recognize the existing and evolving physiological derangements, compounded further by surgical insult, is catastrophic. Discretion is needed more than unwarranted valor and exaggerated belief in your technical ability. Dismissiveness of the other forces working against you is likely to be a source of immense harm to the patient. Ignorance is bliss, whereas knowledge and experience make one a coward. It is better to be a coward when you're dealing with precious human lives.

He Who Fights and Runs Away
May Live to Fight Another Day

Eternal belief in this dictum in surgery will save you a lot of heartache, and it will save lots of lives. There are many situations in surgery in which a tactical retreat can win a lost battle. Surgery is no less than war schemes: strategy, planning, preparedness, timing, not underestimating one's enemy, and choosing the best weapons and soldiers.

The whole concept of damage-control surgery[14] is based on this dictum. Do what is absolutely essential; control the hemorrhage and contamination in a polytrauma patient who is in a lethal physiological state. He or she will not be able to endure the insult of surgical trauma from reconstruction and definitive procedures. Make a hasty retreat to come back another day, better prepared and in better shape to fight it out. There is no point in coming out and telling the relatives that you did everything you could and that you fixed everything but that

---

14   Michael Rotondo et al., "Damage Control: An Approach for Improved Survival in Exsanguinating Penetrating Abdominal Injury," *Journal of Trauma-Injury Infection & Critical Care* 33, no. 1 (1992): 161–167.

unfortunately you could not save the patient because he or she had very bad injuries. This is a common story still echoing in operating room corridors during the debriefing of families. Again, hubris stems from the deep belief in your unfailing ability to perform something and the failure to ask yourself whether it was appropriate to do it and what the consequences could be of pursuing it further.

There are many other situations in surgery in which it is prudent to do the absolute minimum required to save the day. Tuberculous abdomen in endemic places is a prime example where people have tried to be heroic in entering a plastered abdomen with widespread peritoneal disease. The bowel is so friable that wherever one puts a finger, one only makes an iatrogenic hole. The consequences are horrific, leading to the formation of multiple fistulas. It is common to see these often-young patients dying of sepsis with a benign, treatable disease. All this, when all you needed to do was close the abdomen and put them on IV anti-TB and total parental nutrition for six to eight weeks. After this, if you need to go in again for any stricture formation, you will surely be surprised to see what seems to be a totally different belly.

Polytrauma patients are mostly comanaged by a multidisciplinary team. The patients are often under general surgeons and being concurrently looked after by neurosurgeons and orthopedic surgeons. This is the most common combination, but at times, there are more or different combinations. It is your responsibility as a primary team to prioritize management. There will always be pressures from other teams to operate on their bit, but if you feel the patient is unstable and will not be able to tolerate any more insult, let them wait. There is no urgency to fix a fracture or do something else that can safely wait. However, it is not always easy to make this decision.

I once had a young patient who, in addition to a head, chest, and abdominal injury, also had bad compound fractures of the lower limbs. While we were struggling to salvage this patient, the orthopedic surgeons were concerned about his legs. They were pushing us to allow the patient to be taken for debridement. When I told them that the patient was unstable and not ready for any further insult and that he might even die of other injuries, they asked me, "What if he survives?" Sometimes, you are doomed if you do and doomed if you don't. However, the decisions must be well calculated to choose the less harmful option with appropriate timing.

In tertiary-care centers, you receive patients who have had complications of surgery done elsewhere. The transfers are often of very sick patients, usually with sepsis and iatrogenic injuries, enterocutaneous fistulas, or bile-duct injuries. They come in for the long haul and undergo multiple operating room visits, but still, outcomes cannot be guaranteed. It is not easy, and this is why it is important for peripheral hospitals to take on only what they can handle or else refer.

Do it right the first time. Complications can happen in the best of hands. If things have gone wrong and you suspect something abnormal, just shout for help immediately. It doesn't matter if it's a false alarm. If the complications have surfaced afterward in the postoperative phase, then refer them early. Don't cause more harm by remaining in denial or sitting on them doing cosmetic or dubious interventions. It is not fair to the patient, and it is also not fair to make delayed referrals to other colleagues.

There are other less dramatic situations, but still, jumping in is suicidal. It is prudent to select lesser, more conservative options in such cases, too. For patients with enterocutaneous fistulas not manifesting overt sepsis, establish good external drainage and make them into controlled fistulas. Just save the day, and remember that most fistulas close as long as there is no distal obstruction. The very few that don't close can be dealt with later.

I once had a patient who came in hemodynamically unstable, with multiple high-velocity firearm injuries to his face, left chest, and abdomen. The airway was secured, a left chest tube inserted, and a laparotomy performed. This required a quick splenectomy, a left nephrectomy, and exteriorization of the shattered sigmoid colon. There was a lot of bruising in the left retroperitoneal area, and one of the exit wounds was just behind the descending colon.

We mobilized and had a good look, and there was no leak. However, the whole wall longitudinally on the posterior aspect had a hematoma. We did not do anything; we were not planning to do any fancy resection and repairs in such an unstable patient. The stoma was distal to this bruised area. When the stoma started functioning, a couple days later, some stool started coming out of the exit wound in the left lumbar area. We knew that either we had missed the descending-colon injury or there was delayed necrosis due to heat and friction injuries. We did nothing and placed a stoma bag on it, and when the stool became more solid, we kept dressing the wound until it closed.

We all know that emergency surgery has its attendant risks. But some things cannot wait and must be dealt with as an emergency. However, there are many who may come in as an emergency but can be converted into an elective operation by carefully handling them with minimally invasive interventions (such as detorting a sigmoid volvulus and performing elective surgery). This can avoid the need for a stoma and the attendant risks of emergency surgery. Wherever one can safely delay a procedure, one must. It always helps to optimize the patient's condition and prepare the patient to be operated on in the light of day, when the A-team is available, along with all the other help and support available during working hours. Always think carefully, and weigh all options in order to maximize benefit and minimize harm.

The message is to only do what is essential in sick, elderly, septic, and hemodynamically unstable patients. Leave the primary pathology or fancy reconstructions and repairs until another day in these cases. Resecting the pathology and restoring the anatomy may kill the patient. As always, remember that physiology is king and that it is what kills before anything else.

Five

Never Be Cavalier with Somebody Else's Life

~

Entrustment

A sixty-five-year-old patient with a perforated duodenal ulcer and peritonitis who also had COPD and arthritis underwent a laparotomy. Most surgeons would just patch the hole, wash out, and close. Today, we have effective medical options to control the acid output; hence, there is no need to achieve surgical control. But this patient's surgeon, in his own wisdom, decided to do a Billroth II gastrectomy. The patient developed surgical complications and had multiple revisits to operating room, and he eventually succumbed. This is a prime example of being cavalier with somebody else's life.

Patients trust surgeons with their most precious asset: their life. We must be trustworthy and must honor and respect this trust. But what does this actually mean? A trusting relationship first and foremost requires professional integrity with the triangle of medical professionalism—competence, character, and compassion. If you do not have these traits, then you are being cavalier with someone else's life. You are likely to cause harm, and you are not worthy of trust.

Surgical competence is a complex phenomenon, and many factors influence this domain. The worst thing is that it is not a constant; one may be competent in something today but may not be tomorrow for a variety of reasons. However, surgical competence could be defined as having the current knowledge and skills to successfully and safely prepare and perform a task to fruition. One just has to be competent—not necessarily an expert. This has crucial bearing on the outcomes. Incompetence is likely to be a source of serious harm. It is one's moral duty to always remain familiar with the current practices and procedures of one's specialty. Character demands that if you are not up to speed, you must be up-front with the patient. It is obligatory to then refer the patient to somebody else. This should be done purely on the basis of the other person's competence and with no other motive. You must seek help and advice if you are in trouble, instead of compromising patient safety. All of this reflects compassionate care.

There is enough personal experience and literature available to suggest that patients who are voiceless members of society—those who are poor or have no insurance, those from certain ethnic backgrounds, or those who have diminished mental capacity—are all vulnerable. When dealing with such patients, seniors have a very low threshold for delegating patient care to trainees and even leaving them unsupervised. Even juniors have little hesitancy or moral distress in assuming a central role in the care of such patients.

Academic tertiary-care centers have high populations of sick and complex patients. It is challenging for them to provide experience and exposure to trainees in routine stuff. In order to get good routine volumes and case mix, these centers are frequently accessing free public-sector facilities for their trainees in resource-poor settings. There is no dearth of patients and diseases at these places. The staff and resources are unable to cope. They are inundated with work, and the poor patients are suffering. The patients are not interested in *who* will operate on them; they are begging and asking, "*When* will somebody operate on me?" This makes them vulnerable and exposes them to exploitation. These places become training grounds for novices who are left totally unsupervised. This is very sad. The worst thing is that there is very little remorse among the trainers and trainees.

This attitude toward vulnerable populations challenges the moral foundation of surgery's code of ethics. This should never be allowed to happen. Each life is equally precious and entrusted to you—rich or poor, young or old—regardless of color or creed. Everyone deserves the same attention and treatment based on medical needs and no other factors. Training programs must ensure that trainers and trainees never violate patient trust. Any trust-violating tendencies must be observed and nipped in the bud early. Always work within your competencies, with appropriate supervision when needed.

Every patient, every disease, and every operation must get the same care, concentration, and attention to detail. Get it right the first time rather than chase complications. It pays to be paranoid about every resection, every tie, every transfixed vessel, every suture placed, every anastomosis, and every iatrogenic hole closed. There is no room for cutting corners; it is better to be safe than sorry. This doesn't mean that trainers must do everything themselves. Just ensure that things are done to your satisfaction, as you would have done them, without compromising patient safety. However, if you need to take over at any point, you must. At the end of the day, the patient's life is entrusted foremost to you.

It is also a fallacy to assume that one's number of years of training correlates with expected competencies. Individual residents within a training year are incomparable in many ways, and that is true for their skills development, too. Know your residents well; give them only what they can handle, or supervise them. It is also important for their confidence and development that somebody observes them, takes them through a procedure, and gives them good feedback.

It is now common knowledge that there is increased morbidity and even mortality with many near misses during the changing-of-the-guard period at hospitals. This happens every year when new inductees join and juniors are promoted to their next levels. All over and at all levels, there is chaos, like an earthquake. The tremors are particularly felt in surgery.

Already, many things, like better orientation programs, have been put in place to minimize the damage. Still, a word for trainers and trainees: It is not acceptable—morally, ethically, professionally, or by any standards—for anybody to become a victim of such an administrative upheaval. There must be a very low threshold for seeking advice; double-check everything. Faculty must watch things like a hawk and be available both physically and by any means of communication to support this phase of transition.

In this entrusting relationship, there is no allowance for anybody to be cavalier with somebody else's life. Everyone should work within the accepted norms of practice, competence, and personal limitation. Otherwise, refer or consult, but never mess around with other people's lives.

Value Judgments

Historically, surgeons have performed mutilating surgeries, commando operations, extended radical mastectomies, hemicorporectomies, forequarter amputations, pelvic exenterations, and so on. All these heroic operations requiring massive tissue excisions for broadly invasive malignancies (primary and/or metastasis) were done regularly. These were all done in good faith with a license to practice the mind-set of the prevailing understanding and craft of the times.

There was little attention paid to tumor biology and behavior, the quality of life, cost-benefit analysis, and potential for infections and other comorbidities. Human physical, physiological, psychological, and social endurance were tested to the limits. If it could be technically done, it was done without even blinking. One still sees patients who have undergone commando operations covering the operated sides of their faces with an extended headscarf because they know their faces would scare people away.

It's all about making value judgments between the quality and the quantity of life. However, the *quality of life* is such an emotive subject that whenever one broaches it, the debates become emotionally charged and ethically complex. One school of thought believes that the concept of the quality of life should not be used because it undermines the intrinsic dignity and worth of human life. This view may have some merit; it stems from the strong view that human life is not a commodity and should not be subjected to any value judgments. However, the quality of life has very wide and universal philosophical, political, and health-related implications. We are talking about the quality of life as a goal of health care. This is a multidimensional concept that aims to preserve physical, mental, emotional, and social well-being. As a natural extension of this, the quality of life should be the goal of surgical care, too.

Because it is an intervention-based specialty, surgery poses many challenges, especially in cancer care and end-of-life decisions. Today, we have the knowledge, technology, and skills to perform interventions to prolong life and achieve some goals of care in the interim. But what quality of life are we preserving and at what cost? The cost is not necessarily in terms of money but more in terms of physical, social, and psychological endurance. In this sense, the quality of life becomes a benchmark for guiding human activity. It lends itself to a concept of *assessment and evaluation.* There are many evaluation tools available. Unfortunately, one notices that the evaluations are directed primarily by the caregivers and the caregiving processes. The patients and families do partake in these discussions, but caregivers heavily influence the decisions. This is obvious and common in resource-poor settings.

The other issue is about our deep conviction in what we practice and subject our patients to—our prevailing dogma. What we forget is that given the way surgical science is advancing, probably 50 percent of whatever we practice today is likely to become obsolete in ten years. Unfortunately, what we don't know is which 50 percent. This is particularly happening in recent times due to our better understanding and micro-level appreciation of the basis of disease manifestations. In many areas, this understanding has completely changed the theory and practice of surgery. Unfortunately, many people who challenged the prevailing dogmas of their times suffered ridicule until they were vindicated.

It was only in the mid-1950s that George Cryle Jr. (1907–1992),[15] the famous American surgeon, first challenged the idea in cancer surgery that "More is better." His opinion stirred the pot; it was purely based on his academic foresight and observation, but it brought the discourse from the academic echelons to the public forums. His philosophy was later supported by scientific evidence discovered by Bernard Fisher[16] and a research group who did randomized-control trials in early breast cancer and showed no difference in survival with radical mastectomy versus breast conservation plus radiotherapy. Today, we have the means to do anything possible to prolong life, and the motto has changed to "Less is better," all due to a fundamental acceptance that tumor biology is king.[17]

Yet again, the entire concept and philosophy of surgery in my career has made a total U-turn due to appreciation that physiology is king. In the early days of my career, we were told things like "Big surgeons make big cuts," "Don't operate through keyholes," "Never compromise your exposure or access," and "A fourteen-inch wound heals equally as well as a four-inch wound." Today, it is all about less, smaller, and minimally invasive simply because we have become aware after many painful lessons that physiology is king. There is a realization that minimal metabolic and endocrine response to surgical injury and insult is better.

Cancer today is viewed as a systemic disease most of the time at presentation, and here, tumor biology is king. Therefore, more thoughtful, carefully planned, and individualized multidisciplinary care is required.

All these historical retreats from the mind-sets of past practices should be enough to bring some humility to the current practices and proceedings. One needs to first and foremost acknowledge the limitations

---

15 Wolfgang Saxon, "Dr. George Crile Jr., 84, Foe of Unneeded Surgery, Dies," *The New York Times*, September 12, 1992.

16 "Bernard Fisher Reflects on a Half-Century's Worth of Breast Cancer Research," *Journal of the National Cancer Institute* 97, no. 22 (November 2005): 1636–1637.

17 Cady Blake, "Principles in Surgical Oncology," *Archives of Surgery* 132, no. 4 (April 1997): 338–346.

of one's current understanding of things. This attitude has far-reaching implications for achieving the goals of surgical care and influencing decisions about quality-of-life issues.

In comparison, the practice of surgery in resource-poor settings is dissociated from issues of the quality of life. The context, values, and challenges are different and complex for our patients. The care and remedies for the patients are not dictated by what *should* be done but by what *can* be done within the constraints of resource-poor settings. There is no luxury of choice here about the quality of life. Due to poor access to human and material resources, we are still practicing the surgical mind-set of the last century.

For example, even the few patients who present with early breast cancer cannot be offered breast conservation because many places have no access or cannot afford to have radiotherapy, and these patients all get modified radical mastectomy. A lower quality of life is accepted to improve survival rates and sometimes to save costs. Forget about anybody even thinking of immediate or delayed breast reconstruction in such patients, even if it is available. Poor patients have difficulty accessing open surgery; how can they even dream of having minimally invasive surgery? Even patients with low rectal cancer where a sphincter can be saved get an abdominoperineal resection (APR) and a permanent stoma. This is because circular and transverse stapling devices are prohibitively expensive or not available or there is no expertise in using them.

It is also not easy to predict in such settings how values and beliefs influence people when making difficult value judgments between quality and quantity. I once had a thirty-eight-year-old man with a poorly differentiated, seemingly early, and very low rectal cancer. He was told that he needed to have his rectum removed with a permanent colostomy. After this major operation, depending on the pathological stage, he would probably be given chemo and radiation therapy.

The patient asked, "Will I be cured then?"

I told him, "It depends on the stage," and I gave him a tentative prognosis based on his age and the tumor biology.

He said, "I would rather die than have a permanent colostomy. Let me enjoy the little time I have left in peace."

Five months later, I saw him, totally emaciated and completely obstructed, being prepared for a diverting stoma. He had no regrets.

The majority of patient decisions in resource-poor settings are influenced by financial constraints. Unfortunately, patients do not spell them out because of self-respect and dignity. What would a patient do with a permanent colostomy if he or she cannot afford to buy a colostomy bag for a day, let alone for life? The cost of a colostomy bag today is four to five times the daily wage of an unskilled worker. The question for such patients is whether to feed their hungry children or buy a colostomy bag for themselves.

Many a time, I would finish an outpatient clinic in a public-sector hospital and find a few sick patients still lying around in the outpatient area on benches or even on the floor with relatives comforting them. In an effort to assist them, you discover that you had already seen them in clinic and given them admission slips. Upon you inquiring about why the patient has not been admitted, the relative is quiet until a bystander tells you that they don't have ten rupees (less than ten cents) to pay for the admission fee. This is at least a salvageable situation as you could afford to pay for the few lying there, but I always wondered about the patients who were quietly taken away instead of facing further indignity and dishonor. This is a tough and unforgiving environment in which human suffering and quality-of-life issues have little influence in the overall scheme of things.

Despite the massive limitations in resource-poor settings, the principles around the world must be the same. The quality of life after any intervention needs to be central to every discussion about the care plan. I can obtain consent for virtually anything; this is dependent on how much I conceal and how much I reveal. But is this medicine, and is it ethical? We must be up-front about the quality of life, and physician perceptions should not influence such decisions. The quality of life has to be the patient's decision, and it can only be made if patients are given full and informed choices. Who are we to decide about the individual value judgments between quality versus quantity? We need to understand what each patient values more.

Twilight of Life

Surgery is a discipline in which it is crucial to have conviction in what you are doing. One could argue that this is true for anything in life. But because surgery is invasive and risky, it is incumbent on us to choose well and act with conviction. Such decisions have financial and resource implications as well; however, it is all easier said than done.

In the early '80s, during my training in England, half of the surgical emergencies were poor, moribund patients from geriatric wards with perforated diverticular disease, perforated or bleeding peptic ulcers, obstructed colon cancer, and so on. It was so sad because the majority of these patients had multiple comorbidities; they were deaf, senile, demented, and unaware of the world around them. They were just waiting to die of something. Now suddenly, there was an acute surgical emergency, and there was an expectation all around that something should be done. How can you let somebody die? Surgeons are supposed to preserve life. Contrary views were considered inhumane and unethical.

When I brought some (not all) of these patients to the operating room, I was faced with another big hurdle I had to cross. One of our very senior consultant anesthetists, who somehow invariably was on call with me, asked, "Why do you want to operate on this patient, young man?" This is when his resident had already done a preoperative review and had already briefed him about it. He still made sure to challenge me morally every time about my decision. I explained that the patient had peritonitis and that he would surely die if I didn't do anything. Very annoyingly, the anesthetist said, "My friend, he will die anyway whether you do or don't do anything. But why do you want me to be an accomplice to murder? Don't you dare do anything to me when I am at this age and in this state of life—just let me go!"

More than thirty-five years down the road, nothing much has changed. The question still haunts me as to when and where to draw the line. Just recently, I had two patients who epitomize the predicament we all face, even today.

The first one was a ninety-six-year-old lady who presented with an acute abdomen with perforated DU due to the use of nonsteroidal anti-inflammatory drugs (NSAID) for joint pain. I always say that age is not a number; one can have a forty-year-old decrepit and a ninety-six-year-old spring chicken. Our lady did not have any significant comorbidity; she was ambulant around the house, and she was even doing all her small daily chores for herself. Upon examination, she was a pleasant lady who was fully alert and compos mentis. She had tachycardia, tachypnea, low urine output, and peritonitis. She also had a huge incisional hernia from a sixty-year-old right paramedian scar. All her children had died, and she was living with and being looked after by her three very loving grandsons. They did not even know she had a hernia or what surgery had been done.

I had a meeting with the grandchildren and explained to them that she was elderly and that all her organs had done their time. Such people may look well. But they are living on the edge, and any insult just tips them over like dominos. She also had this huge hernia, the reduction of which was likely to produce compartment syndrome, and I could not avoid dealing with it. I had to find a way to house the contents somewhere, somehow. In that contaminated surgery, I could only do a tissue repair, which would not be effective.

They asked, "What are her chances if we do or don't do anything?" I said that either way, she would die, but there was a very remote chance that she might live if we operated on her. It was a mistake to say this. I have been in trouble many times before because of that statement, but I cannot help being factual. They just latched onto that ray of hope and asked us to go all the way. I tried to dissuade them, but they had made up their minds. I knew they were doing it for the sake of their departed parents. During the discussion, they had said that she was the only living memory of their parents. I asked the patient as well, and she went with the grandchildren's decision.

We operated with no conviction, but we did what we would have done had we thought she was going to survive. We had to first handle the hernia to enter the belly, and then we did the absolute minimum necessary. She was initially very sick in the intensive-care unit (ICU)—intubated, ventilated, and on inotropes, with multiorgan dysfunction. But slowly and gradually, she started getting better. She came off everything, including the ventilator, and was now only on noninvasive ventilation at night. She was tolerating nasogastric-tube (NGT) feeds and even communicated to the family, and we thought that this was a miracle. Then one day, she just gave up. With no rhyme or reason, with every parameter near normal, she died peacefully on the sixteenth post-op day. We already had consent for do not resuscitate (DNR). Our chief resident said, "It seems she only came back to say goodbye to everybody."

The second patient was an eighty-eight-year-old lady who was well and active previously. She developed acute cholecystitis for which she had a laparoscopic cholecystectomy in another city. She went into retention once the catheter was removed, and she had a recent history of several episodes of urinary-tract infection (UTI). The urologist there decided to take her back to the operating room for a cystoscopy forty-eight hours after the initial surgery. She suffered a post-op myocardial infarction (MI) after this intervention and was shifted to our hospital under the interventional cardiologist and admitted to the coronary-care unit (CCU).

While she was in the CCU, I was asked to review her postoperative status. She was also complaining of increased frequency of stools—not loose and no blood but with a frequency of twice daily. There was no associated abdominal pain; on examination, she was stable, and the abdomen was appropriate for any similar postoperative patient. A CAT scan had already been done, and it showed post-op changes and extensive diverticular disease of the sigmoid colon. There was some fat stranding around but with no collection. These changes could have been postoperative or due to developing acute diverticulitis. However, she was already on appropriate antibiotics, and this may have masked the clinical signs of infection. We decided to continue conservative management due to her overall condition and especially her cardiac status. We continued appropriate antibiotics to cover the acute diverticulitis just in case.

A week later, she developed a small-bowel intestinal obstruction and manifested signs of sepsis. A CAT scan revealed a small-bowel obstruction with loops adherent in the pelvis. There was now more pronounced fat stranding in the mesentery and around the diverticuli of the sigmoid colon with a small abscess in the pelvis. A diagnosis of complicated diverticulitis was made, and she was prepared for high-risk major surgery: a Hartmann's procedure. The anesthetist, cardiologist, and I were very pessimistic about the outcome. We could do the surgery, and it was indicated, too. But we were also sure that she would not stand it due to her recent MI and cardiovascular instability. We had very little conviction about operating on her.

The family and the patient wanted to go all the way, and they signed the high-risk consent form. She was resuscitated and taken to the OR that same evening. She underwent the release of pelvic adhesions of the small bowel; they were forming the wall of a pelvic abscess, and it was drained. A very quick Hartmann's procedure was done. She was very unstable during surgery due to her very labile, hemodynamic state and almost crashed three times on the table. It was a nightmare for all of us. I kept hearing the anesthetist say, "I am going to lose her anytime." When we finished, she was now on all the works for a critical-care patient; she was also transfused blood as she was very oozy due to antiplatelet medications, and she was given platelets.

Postoperatively, as expected, she was shifted to the ICU; and she had a very stormy course for about seventy-two hours due to the surgery, severe sepsis, and her cardiac condition. She had clear manifestations of multiorgan dysfunction. However, we never gave up, and we continued to support every organ until she made a turnaround. Then we were able to gradually wean her off inotropes and to extubate her, and she made a slow and steady recovery. Eventually, after prolonged hospitalization, she was transferred for rehabilitation and later returned back home to a normal life. It has been more than a year, and she has visited us once from her hometown. I am so glad that she does not want the stoma reversed. In fact, she was ever so grateful to us for resolving her long-standing problem of chronic constipation!

Both these patients were insured and in the private sector. I know that in the public sector, they would not even figure into the scheme of things. This is the most disturbing part of the practice of surgery. As I have already mentioned in another context, if one can afford it, one can influence any health-care decision, conviction or no conviction. This raises huge moral and ethical issues for caregivers in any setting.

Health care, and especially critical care, is very expensive anywhere in the world. In resource-poor settings, it is not only expensive but also a scarce commodity. Time and again, very reluctantly, you are forced into situations where you have very little conviction, but you are still sucked into doing some things that seem like exercises in futility. There are still no clear answers in such situations.

There is another difficult dilemma in which families agree to no surgical intervention but want to continue treating the surgical condition with medical means, such as treating a frank peritonitis with antibiotics. Sometimes, they wish not to escalate therapy, but they don't want de-escalation either. If things get worse, they agree to a DNR. Some clearly indicate no desire for any active intervention and agree to just tender loving care. Does this mean no chronic medications and no blood-sugar management? If they are on a ventilator, does one take the tube out, or what kind of ventilator support should one provide? Does one switch off the monitors and not take any vitals? And even if one monitors vitals, what is the point of monitoring if you are not going to intervene?

There is very little clarity on many such issues; we just continue to take half-hearted measures without much conviction. Sometimes, we do this for the comfort of the family so that they don't feel that their relative is totally abandoned and everybody is now waiting for the inevitable, which is actually true. This period can be prolonged and agonizingly painful for everybody, especially if one continues with such supports as I have mentioned above.

There is plenty of literature around, but it still does not help in real-life situations. Today, the aging population is increasing around the world, especially in the nonindustrialized world. Their presentation with acute surgical emergencies is also on the rise. It is high time to discuss and deliberate on these issues as a society. People need to write advance directives if they do not want to prolong their misery. I have seen time and again families in dilemmas, hesitant to make decisions when hope is fading away and the chances of meaningful recovery are minimal. Their major concern is always that they do not wish to live with the guilt that they pulled the plug too early.[18] This is very tough and heartrending. One always sees families breaking down in tears and in distress when they have agreed to withdraw life support. This suffering and guilt could be minimized if people were encouraged to leave advance directives.

Trainees must appreciate that surgeons need to play a proactive role in discussing and deliberating end-of-life issues with patients and families before intervention while discussing their medical-care plan. Documentation of patient wishes about end-of-life issues is as important as documenting medical care; it avoids strain on scarce resources and unnecessary suffering of both patients and families if and when issues of futility of care arise.

---

18 Elizabeth Reis, "Hoping for a Good Death," *The New York Times*, December 1, 2014, http://well.blogs.nytimes.com/2014/12/01/hoping-for-a-good-death/?_r=0.

Six

Your Attitude, Not Your Aptitude, Will Determine Your Altitude

~

Your attitude, not your aptitude, will determine your altitude.

—Zig Ziglar

Egos to Ethos

Not long ago, cancer patients would receive treatment according to the specialty they first consulted. This still happens in many places. Most commonly, surgeons led the way; they made the diagnosis, evaluated the extent of disease, and, for solid tumors, would perform the most effective surgical therapy. If the patient ended up with a physician, he or she would be investigated and managed or referred on their understanding of the problem and approach. Today, once diagnosis is made about the type and stage of cancer, the patient has options of treatment modalities by medicine, surgery, radiation, nuclear medicine and immunotherapy—alone, in combination, or as sandwich therapies. This requires a multidisciplinary discussion in order to preserve and prolong life in an evidence-based, cost-effective, and minimally invasive way. Current-day cancer care does not allow us to work in individual silos. Other options cannot be an afterthought or any thought at all.

There are two distinct types of multidisciplinary care. Both produce different kinds of challenges. The first kind of multidisciplinary care is when multimodality treatment is needed to treat the same disease. The field of oncology is the commonest example. Cancer treatment requires individual or combination modalities, both in neoadjuvant and adjuvant settings. These cases absolutely must be discussed at multidisciplinary-team (MDT) meetings (tumor boards) prior to any kind of intervention. The agreed-upon management plan for each individual patient must be documented and followed by all caregivers. In the nonindustrialized world, MDTs are uncommon. Where these meetings do happen, it is commonly observed that the discussion surrounds the need for an adjuvant therapy. One intervention has already happened, most commonly surgery. MDT meetings need to happen regularly in all hospitals prior to any intervention to provide evidence-based, holistic, and well-integrated care.

Organizing multidisciplinary meetings of this nature in resource-poor settings can certainly be a big challenge, but it is certainly doable in places where there are human and physical resources available to provide such multidisciplinary care. When this is not possible, prior-agreed protocols should be used. No matter how the patient presents or to which practitioner, they can ensure appropriate standards of care.

The other, more common type of multidisciplinary care is due to the increasing complexity of patients with multiple medical problems. The highly specialized nature and practice of medicine today invariably involves more than one physician in the care of a patient. There are advantages and disadvantages of this compartmentalization and fragmentation of care. The advantage is that an expert specialist treats each ailing system; nobody can be a master of everything. The patient receives focused care, and studies have shown that such an approach has good outcomes. Physicians must also work within their domains due to hospital-credentialing processes and the avoidance of legal issues. It is also a moral and a professional obligation to consult or refer to an expert whenever a patient's needs demand. The disadvantages are that illness is a phenomenon of a sick body and not some system(s). The sick body can be a manifestation of internal pathological processes, of the mind, or of both. Isolated approaches and fragmented care lack a holistic approach to patients' disease manifestations. Unfortunately, the comprehensive internist has become extinct.

This multidisciplinary care is causing problems of ownership of the patient and issues of continuity of care. The major challenge being faced is poor communication; it seems that physicians talk to files more and to each other less. These often-illegible notes and orders may never be read unless a physician is particularly looking for them, and all this could have detrimental consequences on patient outcomes. The other issues are of an incoherent team approach and a lack of central focus and coordination. Most often, physicians providing care come at different times, make independent decisions, ask for a new set of investigations, change treatments, write orders, and disappear.

I once walked into our surgical ward and saw my thirty-eight-year-old patient being wheeled out of the HDU. Prior to his current illness, he was a healthy man who was now recovering from severe acute biliary pancreatitis. He had infected necrosis and required pancreatic necrosectomies. I asked them where they were taking him, and they said for an MRI.

"An MRI of what?" I asked. The nurse said that the neurologist had come to see the patient and asked for a head MRI. "Why was the neurologist called to see the patient?" I asked. The junior resident who was with me informed me that in the morning round, the chief resident asked for a consult because the patient was exhibiting fleeting confusional states.

My immediate question was, "Does he have any neurological deficit?" The answer was no. I asked him, "What are the chances of finding something on an MRI? Could this state not be explained by septic metabolic encephalopathy, considering what he has gone through and is still going through?" The resident said that they thought the same, but the chief said it was better to consult, just to be on the safe side.

This example typifies an isolated approach to care, and it magnifies the problem of generating unnecessary consults. Lack of conviction in what you are doing, defensive practice of medicine, and diluting responsibility are prime causes of such practices. Then when one invites in other people unnecessarily and doesn't agree with what they may have to say, this creates even more problems. There are so many egos involved that even if one tries to discuss and reason out things, it is taken as an offense.

I remember a physician once abandoned the patient and walked out on me for discussing his management plan. Human beings are the most difficult and unpredictable beings on this earth. How could one walk away from a patient? Such are the realities and sensitivities of multidisciplinary care. Patients are at the mercy of such care. Upon discharge, a patient invariably receives two to three appointments with different physicians on different days at different times. Who cares for the inconvenience of the sick? Patients unfortunately are getting the worst in this gambit. They long to know, "Who is my doctor?"

Whatever philosophy we may believe in, the reality is that this multidisciplinary care is here and is the future of medicine. People are already specialists of just a single disease or an organ, not even of a system. However, for this system to function appropriately, we need to understand the ethos and obligations of this multidisciplinary practice. There is a need to establish a framework to ensure some rationality in the proceedings.

First and foremost, care must always be patient centered, and we must never forget our moral responsibility to respect the person. It must be understood that the primary team is in charge of the patient; ownership, responsibility, integration, and coordination of care are the duties of this team. Other teams have secondary, consultative, and advisory roles. They are not meant to come and take over the care of the patient and start doing things without engaging the primary team. However, if at any stage the nature and condition of the patient changes, then care should be transferred, with mutual consultation, to any other main caregiver. Decisions must always be made by discussion and consensus. The teams should communicate better and develop methods of evolving consensus by joint rounds and reminders to consult notes and reports. This requires a cultural change from egos to ethos by interdisciplinary cooperation and compromise to avoid conflicts. Disagreements in management should always lead to a respectful exchange of views. Whatever is decided should be in the best interest of the patient.

Disagreements may even exist within the primary-care team, but they must follow the attending physician's orders at all times. This is not meant in any way to kill any debate and discussion about patient condition and management. However, the final word should be that of the attending. This is simply because the patient is his or her responsibility and under his or her care. Given the attending's training, experience, expertise, and much greater responsibility, one needs to follow their orders. The attending physician is ethically and morally responsible and legally liable for the actions of interns, residents, and other caregivers. Therefore, the junior team members conversely have a duty and obligation, to their attending and to the patient, not to act recklessly or without the knowledge and approval of supervisors.

The other issue is of team dynamics within the organization as surgical teams have a very hierarchical structure. In clinical care, there are two tiers or levels of interaction between two sets of providers. One is at the consultant level of different specialties, and this is usually a direct, amicable, and complementary relationship. However, this does not mean that the consultants are angels. There are egos, turf wars, professional rivalries, and, unfortunately, even personal animosities and vendettas. It can become ugly at times. Such people usually don't see eye to eye and never mutually consult each other. Unfortunately, sometimes, one of them may be on call that day or the only one around. No matter what your personal relations may be, they should not affect patient care in any way.

The second tier consists of resident teams of one specialty interacting with other specialty teams; this happens 24/7, and it is a big conundrum. Luckily, it's rarely personal and more often a historical specialty rivalry. I hate to generalize, but by and large, surgical residents have huge egos. They are known to always have a point to prove. Many have an attitude. Wherever they go, they have this uncanny habit of offending. Most often, the skirmishes are with their historical rivals, the physicians. But the other residents are not spared, including those in anesthesia, radiology, and always the emergency department. They look at obstetrics and gynecology (OB-GYN) residents with contempt, as some lesser cousins who always need help and often need to be assisted.

This is unacceptable and should never happen. It is all right to be proud of what one does, but it does not give one a license to become arrogant and demeaning to others. Respecting others and their views will only gain more respect. One needs to learn to command respect. These attitudinal traits in residents need to be curbed early; residents must learn to be team players and team builders. Humility is a virtue that we must all practice if we are to get the best out of people. At times, the issues may be genuine and annoying, but the norms of civilized behavior should still be to praise in public and scold in private. We need to all work together for the best interests of the patients.

Treating Patients as Cases

Medicine is more than a job, and patients are not objects of inquiry. Unfortunately, patients often feel that we are uncaring, impersonal, and dissociated. If we examined this carefully, we would understand that there are many attitude issues among caregivers, and the perceptions of the patients are not far from reality.

I once had a retired senior civil servant—highly educated and a cultured man—under my care for a major cancer procedure. He stayed longer than usual in the hospital because of his comorbidities. He was a quiet and unassuming individual but an astute observer. He visited the clinic much later for a follow-up. I asked him to narrate the human element of his experience of being a patient in the hospital.

He lifted his head up and looked at me with gloomy eyes and a sad smile, and he went into a pensive mood. After a pause, with his persuasive and soft voice, he said, "It was my first-ever hospital experience, and I never thought somebody would ever want to know or care about what I felt."

He was astonished that I had put him into a situation of rewinding the experience he largely wanted to forget. He said, "People don't come to the hospital for a picnic. I learnt why we are called *patients*; it's because we are supposed to be patient and endure suffering and indignity. Isn't that the expectation?"

I knew he was being sarcastic and assured him to candidly speak up because it would be helpful. He hastily added, "The fact that you asked specifically about the human interaction tells me that you know there is a problem."

He was again quiet and pensive and then said, "It is a big problem." He described the interaction at best as cold, dissociated, and indifferent. He was in pain, but the voices—and forget about the body language—of the doctor and the nurse showed no sign of concern. When he pressed the call bell, they would respond in their sweet time and then disappear, only to be seen again at the next call bell. It was as if some object was lying there rather than a human being.

They were always at the counter, either on the phone or busy filling out their paperwork. Whenever they came on their own, they came with a job to do. The doctor had to check the patient out and was more interested in his results, charts, and sheets. The nurse came to look at the drip or do some observations or some other chores. There was no gentleness or care in doing things; even bathing in bed was like bathing some inanimate object. The food tray was left on the patient's table at the foot of the bed for him to figure out how to reach. Besides the ceremonial exchange, nobody cared to smile, look him in the eyes, or ask him how he was. They need to understand to *empathize* and not *sympathize* with the suffering of their patients. It made him feel very helpless and at the mercy of people who did not exhibit much mercy. He said, "I would be their father's age to your young doctors, but I did not even get a dignified human exchange worthy of even that relationship."

He said that the rounds of the team should be observed because there is no privacy or confidentiality about them. At the end of the ward round, every patient on the ward would know his diagnosis, his progress, and even whether he had passed flatus or passed a stool. He stated that this was embarrassing and dehumanizing. They need to also be sensitive of what theoretical discussions they have at the bedside of the patient. Not everybody understands everything or the extent to which it could be alarming for some patients. In the end, he said, "There needs to be more care, empathy, dignity, and respect for the human beings lying on your ward beds."

The above case exemplifies the stories of many patients I have interviewed over the years. The other common observation of patients is the perception of being an object of interest or inquisition: "Oh, that fifty-nine-year-old on bed twenty-five is a beautiful case and a classical presentation of obstructive jaundice due to carcinoma head of the pancreas. You must go and see him before he gets operated on tomorrow."

Patients feel that caregivers neither want nor even try to make the human connections necessary to empathize with their suffering. There is reasonable validity in these perceptions. Many doctors relate to patients as bed numbers, surgical diagnoses, procedures, and even some other self-awarded titles. This is undignified and indecorous conduct.

We need to understand that patients are not mere cases; they are human beings with dignity, emotions, and feelings. During sickness and suffering, they become more sensitive to trivial issues. Caregivers must be conscious of this fragile emotional state and make allowance for patient expectations. It may be relevant here to also reflect on the concept of *human dignity*, on the idea that a human being has an innate right to be valued and respected and to receive ethical treatment. Human dignity is beyond the boundaries of color, class, or creed, and it signifies the intrinsic worth of human life. We must respect and uphold the dignity and worth of human life at all times.

Custodians of Information

Physicians become custodians of a lot of personal and health-related information. Confidentiality of this patient information is almost absolute, barring few exceptions. In such cases, one may have a legal reporting obligation, such as when there is risk to other peoples' lives (as in cases of communicable diseases).

Patients not only trust their doctors with all their personal information but also lay bare their modesty to a virtually unknown person. This is a very sensitive and personal matter. Any disclosure of this information would be detrimental to patient interests and destroy trust in doctors. We all need to be very conscious of this role and responsibility and guard this information religiously at all times. One must be always aware of the many interested parties to this information, and it should only be divulged with patient consent and after due diligence.

Unfortunately, the general perception and observation is that we are too casual about the sensitivity of this information. This is an attitudinal issue among caregivers, and it is exacerbated by several other factors that may be directly or indirectly responsible for these perceptions. Let's just focus on the trainees and examine the commonly observed loose talk that happens at that level. One just needs to quietly listen and observe residents, interns, and students in hospital elevators, corridors, lounges, and cafeterias. One will hear patient stories and their findings being openly discussed in the presence of the public. I believe that this is not ill-intended but ill-mannered. It is out of ignorance toward the sensitivity of information and the implications of their behavior.

Then there is social media, which has surpassed all boundaries and limitations. Patient-related material, pictures, and information are on social media in no time. I was once sent a link on Facebook, and when I opened it, I found one of the goriest images I had ever seen. It was a posed picture of our chief resident in neurosurgery with a patient on the operating table. The head of the patient was visible, with a craniotomy wound and exposed brain and a lot of blood and irrigation fluid on the drapes and even dripping on the floor. This was taken after evacuating a large extradural hematoma. It was like a hunter posing with his kill. The caption below said, "This is how I make my living."

The comments of his friends were even more sickening. He was asked by the program director to immediately remove the picture and was summoned to explain. He was obviously very ashamed and full of remorse. When I asked him how he could do such a thing, he said that he thought that since the patient was not identifiable, it was all right. He never considered the broader implications of such irresponsible conduct. It again boils down to the issue of respect and appreciation of human life and dignity. It has to be profoundly sacrosanct to all of us and should never be made an object of mockery or scorn. We need to seriously assimilate and espouse these values as health-care professionals.

The other biggest threat today to patient information and privacy comes from electronic medical records and access to all online data from ancillary services. This data is available at the touch of a button from any hospital computer, and it can be remotely accessed anywhere. The passwords are not restrictive to any direct health-care provider; once one has it, one has access to any information, whether one needs it or not. As a surgeon, I can access even the records of a psychiatric patient or laboratory reports from the HIV clinic.

In addition, passwords are passed around very casually, mostly to expedite things rather than with any malicious intent. There are often no proper log-outs by users, and one may have left the computer a long time before it automatically logs out. The sense of responsibility and sensitivity of information needed to be a custodian of such information is considerable. This is becoming a huge menace, and there are currently no clear answers as to where and how it will end. Certainly, electronic records and reports have made life very easy, resulting in speed, accessibility, and reduced costs. But until the dust settles down, we all need to be conscious of the confidentiality of patient information and exhibit more responsible behavior.

Fortunately, advancements are occurring, although not yet widely available, where electronic-solutions passwords can be issued only to those with a right to know. This can be readily screened so that senior staff can be informed when electronic health records are searched by those not entitled.

Confidentiality is a major pillar of the trust-based patient-doctor relationship. The betrayal of patient trust at any time is detrimental for caregivers and the caregiving processes. Therefore, respect the privacy of all gathered patient information during provision of care; protect its confidentiality at all costs, at all levels, and by all caregivers.

Seven

When You Have Nothing,
You Have Nothing to Lose

~

Resource-Poor Settings

For a surgeon, the most challenging world is the third world, where the majority of the world population resides. It is riddled with poverty and disease, with few resources and limited access to health care. Hospitals, clinics, medical surgical supplies, technology, and human resources are scarce. Patients are suffering, and some die of acute, curable diseases due to the lack of timely access. Others with chronic diseases die while waiting to be treated because their conditions worsen when there is not much hope left of a cure.

The Lancet Commission on Global Surgery 2015 report states that five billion people around the world do not have access to surgery and anesthesia care. Access is worst in low-income and lower-middle-income countries, where nine of ten people cannot access basic surgical care. An additional 143 million procedures are needed each year to save lives and prevent disability.[19] This is a sad and painful state of affairs, and it is not surprising that surgeons working in such environments must struggle relentlessly with every aspect of surgical care.

Arthur Ashe once said, "Start where you are; use what you have; do what you can." The life of a surgeon in resource-poor settings around the world is nothing but this, all the time. If one waits for the luxuries available to surgeons in the developed world, one will never be able to do anything significant. Even dreams are not affordable. This does not in any way mean that one can cut corners or compromise the safety of patients in the name of a lack of resources. That is neither innovative nor acceptable. It is actually innovative to produce equally good outcomes with whatever one has by improvising in the context in which one is working. Despite everything, there is a lot one can achieve and a lot of good work one can do as long as one is prepared and determined to persevere and innovate.

In early 1990, I had just returned from the West, and I was full of high tech and high talk. I looked at things and the way they were being done with contempt and obvious displeasure. But a few humbling experiences were enough to bring humility to my proceedings and provoke great respect for all that was happening around me.

One day, I was called for help in an emergency encountered by a surgeon in a small, charitable community hospital. He had done a difficult open cholecystectomy and removed a chronic fibrotic gallbladder packed with stones. There was brisk hemorrhage after removal of the gallbladder, and he packed it. He rechecked after a while. The hemorrhage was still brisk, and he could not see the source. He packed it again and called for emergency help.

I went there and found the setup to be even more primitive than anything I had seen before. I discovered a small hole in the portal vein, which happened during dissection, and I asked for a Satinsky clamp.

---

19 John G. Meara et al., "Global Surgery 2030: Evidence and Solutions for Achieving Health, Welfare, and Economic Development," *Lancet* 386 (2015): 569–624.

Everybody was quiet. I asked if they had a bulldog clamp or any vascular instruments. The silence was deafening. I just pinched the hole in the portal vein and put a soft intestinal clamp across the porta hepatis.

I then asked the ancient-looking and very composed male scrub technician, who I think knew well what I was going to ask next, "Do you have a 4/0 prolene suture?" He denied by shaking his head.

I said, "Do you have 5/0 or 3/0 or any fine monofilament, nonabsorbable suture on a sixteen- or eighteen-millimeter needle?"

He did not answer but leaped across to the other trolley and showed me a 2/0 chromic catgut on a thirty-millimeter needle in a glass tube with a fluid preservative and No. 2 silk on a spool! "This is what I have. You can pick and choose."

I looked at the host surgeon in disbelief and was contemplating what to do. I noticed this old tech with thick aphacic glasses unbraiding the No.2 silk on the spool. He pulled out one of the finest filaments from it. Then he asked the runner to get him the box of needles. The runner brought a small steel case and opened it in front of him. It had a sponge to fit the box, and it was soaked in what was probably Cidex. The sponge had many eye needles of different sizes pinned on it. He picked a needle that would match a sixteen-millimeter needle. He threaded that fine filament of silk through the eye and gave it to me on a needle holder. I was dumbfounded by his ingenuity. It was enough to shut up the arrogance of a young surgeon looking around at everything and everybody with contempt. I very quietly and sheepishly repaired the vein, and all went well.

After we descrubbed, I met and praised the tech, thanking him profoundly and expressing a lot of respect, and I asked him about his background. He said he was the senior scrub tech in OBGYN operating rooms in the same teaching hospital where I worked. On his off days and off hours, he worked in smaller hospitals to boost his income and support his poor family. He said he had heard about a new surgeon who had joined, but he was polite enough not to add the words *ignorant* and *arrogant* to his description of me. This was my first humbling experience, which taught me a lot of respect and appreciation for what people were doing and achieving in such trying circumstances.

When one comes from abroad with a mind-set and fixed ideas, one fails to appreciate the importance of the context in which one is going to work. During my early period, we had so much penetrating trauma due to ethnic and political strife in the city. Sometimes, we would operate all day and night. We saw gunshots, stab wounds, and shrapnel injuries, all in young people; and for every colonic injury, we would exteriorize and form a stoma, following the famous dictum "If in doubt, bring it out."

It was such a mindless exercise that even if there was no doubt, it was still brought out. It had become a rule with no exception. In clinics during follow-ups, these patients were absolutely miserable. The cheapest colostomy bag in those days would cost about five dollars, and their earnings were not more than couple of dollars or less a day. They could not afford a square meal; how could they afford a colostomy bag? They just begged for reversal; the waiting lists were long, and it just prolonged their suffering, both economic and social.

One day, a young cobbler came for a follow-up, and he was proud to show me what he had made. There was a cheap, simple, soft leather belt around his waist with a wide area over the stoma, like the dial of a wristwatch. He had cut a round hole in this wide, elliptical part, exactly the size of the stoma. Beyond the hole, he had made stellate cuts in the leather to pinch the edges of a small, thin, black plastic shopping bag. He had tied the handles of this bag on either side of the stoma belt. This was a very cheap, washable stoma device with cheap, disposable shopping bags. I was impressed and humbled again with the human capacity to innovate in times of desperate need. He got lot of work from me as I sent many patients with stomas to him.

The huge morbidity and economic plight resulting from this indiscriminate practice of stoma formation made me question our practice. In our unit, we developed a protocol for selective stoma formation in trauma patients. We created an exception to the rule by doing it only in patients who were elderly and exhibited comorbidities, multiple organ injuries, poor physiological states, gross contamination, and delayed presentation. For patients who were young and hemodynamically stable and presented within four hours with isolated bowel injury or minimal to moderate contamination, we did a primary anastomosis. Every operation was conducted or supervised by an experienced surgeon. We watched the ones with primary anastomosis like a hawk, and we had a low threshold to exteriorize at the earliest sign of trouble.

We managed to reduce unnecessary stoma formation by almost 60 percent, and we achieved a less-than-10-percent leak rate with no mortality. We were ecstatic; this was no small success in the context in which we were working. We tried to publish our small case series in some reputable journals, but it was returned with contemptuous remarks, probably because it challenged the prevailing dogma of that era or simply because it was not their problem. I am glad that today, it is an acceptable practice worldwide, which actually came out of necessity for us.

As one cannot survive otherwise in such resource-poor settings, there are many examples of ingenuity and improvisation: using insulin syringes as colostomy bridges instead of expensive, nonavailable glass rods or plastic flanges; putting pediatric feeding tubes in the lumen of a chest tube and making it into a sump drain for suction and irrigation; using drip set tubes and cutting them into pieces to use as suture splints; and so on.

Resource-poor settings are not just starved for human and physical resources but also suffering due to the low quality of existing human resources. This leads to substandard practices and competency issues, which leads to errors and poor outcomes. However, the patients are mostly simple, illiterate, poor, and very forgiving. They draw strength from their religious beliefs and convictions. They accept many things as fate and destiny ordained by divine wisdom.

Once, a fifty-nine-year-old woman from a village had a core biopsy for a suspicious breast lesion. It was clearly reported without ambiguity as malignant. She underwent a modified radical mastectomy. The final histology report showed no evidence of malignancy. The mistake was terrible and indefensible. On follow-up, the breast surgeon was up-front with the patient and explained that the final report indicated no cancer and that they should not have removed her breast. She immediately knelt and prostrated herself and profoundly thanked God that she did not have cancer. She told the surgeon, "Whatever you did was in my best interest. God has saved me from this terrible disease, and this is a very small price to pay. I am going home with a lot of happiness and prayers for all your team, who looked after me so well."

There are many such examples from working in these settings. Patients have even died due to blatant management errors, and families have walked away with very stoical and fatalistic attitudes. This is a cause for concern because it is human nature that if there is no accountability or consequences, one becomes complacent and accepting of adverse outcomes. Instead of analyzing errors and implementing systems with checks and balances as part of error management, one starts putting the blame for everything on the resource-poor setting. Clearly, many of these things are simple and rectifiable. They do not need any specific or significant resources. One surely needs to reflect on practices in such environments. It is necessary in order to avoid exploitation and to have a greater sense of moral responsibility toward one's patients in these settings.

There are many subspecialty surgical teams that have originated in the West and put up surgical camps all over the developing world. They do a good job, and all come with good intentions. However, due to the lack of local regulatory oversight and the desperation of patients, poor populations are vulnerable to exploitation. Teams should not be allowed to parachute in and jet out, leaving behind patients with no aftercare and little follow-up or long-term rehabilitation. These people are poor and desperate, but they are still human beings who deserve respect and dignified and fair human exchanges. These teams must collaborate with local authorities, agencies, and organizations and ensure that there are, first of all, local capacity-building and training of staff. This is important for patients to be adequately cared for and followed up on once the medical team has gone. It should also be a sustainable development and a mutually beneficial relationship with regular visits and follow-ups.

Trainees and young surgeons in these environments must understand the sheer scale and enormity of the issues and challenges. This can be very overwhelming and at times frustrating, especially when one cannot see any light at the end of the tunnel. It may seem like a perpetual slog with no hope of respite. Burnout in such environments is also common. Despite all these challenges, I can assure you that you can survive and with pride, as did your predecessors.

This survival drive and motivation comes from a deep belief and conviction in the intrinsic value and worth of one's work, something that inherently sounds and feels right and gives immense satisfaction. There is nothing more rewarding than bringing a smile to the face of a suffering, poor human being or than seeing the immense gratitude and tears in the eyes of a poor mother whose child was saved after a bad trauma or the enormous appreciation and indebtedness of many poor patients who received care despite having nothing to give one except prayers. This phenomenon is difficult for one to even comprehend or appreciate unless one works in these conditions and actually experiences them. This is what keeps one going and will keep you all going as young surgeons.

At the end of the day, one needs to appreciate that without pain, one will never understand the meaning of joy. The joy and the immense satisfaction of innovation, improvisation, and developing fair systems and other small successes in improving patient care and outcomes are rewarding beyond imagination. Despite all the frustrations and constraints of this wretched and unfair world, I would still never trade anything for the joy, deep contentment, and sense of accomplishment that I experience in such difficult and trying circumstances.

Justice as Fairness

In medicine, justice is all about fairness. John Rawls (1921–2002), a renowned philosopher of the last century, claimed that "Justice is the first virtue of social institutions, as truth is of system of thought. Justice can be thought of as distinct from and more fundamental than benevolence, charity, mercy, generosity, or compassion."[20] In other words, if one is not fair as an individual, an institution, or as a society, then one cannot espouse nor do justice to any of the other basic ethical values or tenets. One cannot be unfair to someone and yet claim to be merciful or caring.

Justice in health care means accountability in dispensation of health-care resources without any form of discrimination on any basis—distributive justice. It is a very fundamental expectation, and one cannot move forward with any other values unless one develops fair health systems. This value is most often well catered to in the developed world, where resources are plentiful and systems are well developed. By and large, the systems are fair, and distribution is without any discrimination and with accountability at all levels. These systems even allow aggrieved individuals or groups to demand transparency and recourse for any alleged unfairness or wrongdoing. Sadly, however, in many well-developed nations, disparities in care within large cities are all too frequent.

How does one meet the huge challenge of implementing such fair systems across the globe, especially in an inherently unjust world? The third-world gross domestic products (GDPs) are so low, and a meager percentage of them are dedicated to health care despite huge populations with so much disease and poverty. The infamous 10/90 gap[21] of skewed distribution of resources between the developed and developing world is horrible. Imagine what amazing things one could do in less fortunate countries with the cost of a single robot machine being utilized in developed world. The question I ask myself is, how do I practice just medicine in an unjust world?[22] In deprived environments starving for resources, surgeons in some places are made custodians of these meager health-care resources. This is really tough, and it is all the more reason

---

20 John Rawls, "Justice as Fairness: Political Not Metaphysical," *Philosophy and Public Affairs* 14 (Summer 1985): 223–251.

21 "10/90 Gap," Wikipedia, https://en.wikipedia.org/wiki/10/90_gap.

22 "Just Medicine in an Unjust World" (the first International Bioethics Conference, held at Aga Khan University, Karachi, Pakistan; organizing committee chaired by Asad Jamil Raja and members of the Bioethics Group, Aga Khan University, Karachi, Pakistan, 2001).

to understand and appreciate the huge responsibility to develop fair, just, and accountable systems for distributing these pitiful health-care resources.

At the micro level of resource allocation in hospitals, the experience is not encouraging. The claimants are so many, and resources are minimal. There is so much influence and pressure due to overwhelming demands that the disbursement of resources is hardly ever fair. The allocation of scarce funds and limited physical resources—such as general beds, critical-care beds, operating room space and time, elective lists, and even order on the lists—is hardly ever based on medical need or on a first-come-first-serve basis. Patients are bumped off operating lists at the drop of a hat if another more influential patient turns up. These dilemmas are common, and we need to develop fair and accountable systems to overcome extraneous pressures, which come to bear on the custodians of such resources. It would be a great help and relief in easing of their moral burden, too.

I once agonized while I sat through a real case-based debate in the West on whether or not one should transplant a liver to a Down's syndrome child. It was like people squabbling over placement on the table of china and silver, for their problem was not food as they had enough food to eat. In the end, I told them that the problems in resource-poor settings were different. We have no food to eat, and if we had it, we would be quite happy to sit on the floor and eat it. When we have a young man who is otherwise well presenting to us with an end-stage liver disease, he is already history. Our health systems would treat five thousand kids with diarrhea and dysentery rather than spend that money on one liver transplant. Priority setting has true meaning in resource-constraint environments. The emphasis and thrust is on simple, acute, and curable diseases, and they have priority over complex, chronic, and incurable diseases. There is no other choice if one has such scarce resources and so many diverse, competing claimants.

A neurosurgeon friend and my classmate in the West always debated with me about the immorality of the utility theory that the ends justify the means. I would impress upon him that in principle, he may be right, but he cannot be so rigid and ignore the context where this theory may be applicable and valuable. In the context of resource-constraint scenarios anywhere around the world, utility prevails in the centuries-old conflict of duty versus utility. In such environments, we unfortunately have strong utilitarian approaches to health-care problems—the aim is to preserve the lives of as many people as possible, period.

On the global scene, it seems that the expectations of fair distribution of health-care resources are merely pipe dreams. Lip service paid to such ideals sounds cynical when the whole system on which this foundation is laid is intrinsically unjust and immoral. Article 25 of the UN's Universal Declaration of Human Rights states that health equity is a basic human right. This article also requires equity in social conditions and other modifiable determinants of health, such as education, clean water, sanitation, and basic living conditions compatible with human existence. Unfortunately, after sixty-nine years, this article has just remained a slogan. The international and national agencies have failed miserably in supporting this expectation of basic human rights.

Every year, there are a lot of ostentatious shows in the name of the poor and their human rights in all major cities and capitals of economic power around the world. These events are full of crocodile tears and the trampling of the dignity of the poor. At the end of all this fanfare and presentations with complex jargon of statistics, the outcome is zero plus zero equals zero. The eight Millennium Development Goals (MDGs) meant to improve the lives of the poorest of the world have fallen short of their set targets. Three of these goals were specific, health-related indicators with a narrow focus. After fifteen years and billions of dollars, there is now realization about the necessity to impact more widely and in a way that it is sustainable. Therefore, we now have seventeen Sustainable Development Goals (SDGs) to be realized by 2030, of which *good health and well-being* is one of the goals. Nothing has changed in my lifetime; if anything, things have gotten worse. Every talk, every sermon, and every slogan seem farcical; they are condescending, unfair, and insulting.

However, there is some solace for people working in such resource-poor environments. We have an identity and many names: third world, nonindustrialized world, developing countries, low- and middle-income countries (LMIC), resource-poor settings, and many others. These terms are all used interchangeably depending on the convenience and needs of the situation. To be fair, this is a genuine effort to give respectability to our status and existence. However, they are still struggling to find the right name to camouflage this mess. What is there in a name anyway? Calling a pauper a king doesn't change his plight.

The reality is that the number of people living below the poverty line is expanding every day around the world. To date, none of these unfortunate countries has moved up into the line of first-class carriages meant for the elite and exclusive. If anything, the line of third-class carriages for the destitute and deprived is expanding. The usual response to this observation is that governments in such places are corrupt and incompetent. Hence the economic powers have gone on to create a web of mostly self-serving nongovernmental organizations (NGOs). What a disaster. I always wonder, with all the real and armchair philosophers around the world, is it too difficult to create something equitable?

Martin McKneally[23] proposes a framework for clinicians to provide optimal care within resource-constrained environments. His main emphasis is on minimizing the use of marginally beneficial tests and interventions, using the least costly treatments to achieve therapeutic goals, treating patients in order of their need and appearance, supporting conservation of health-care resources, avoiding manipulation of the rules of the health-care system to give unfair advantage to your own patients, employing fair and publicly defensible procedures for resolution of conflicting or competing claims, and informing patients of the impact of cost constraints in a humanistic way. This is not easy, but it has to be done as a collective and shared decision-making process with oversight. How valuable this approach would be in developed nations, with their wasteful overdiagnosis, overinvestigation, and overtreatment. How much we could save and redistribute by critical appraisal of the actions of high-income countries.

Let's not grieve too much; we already suffer a lot every day. We cannot cure all the ills of this world, but we can continue to take care of

---

23 Martin McKneally, "Resource Allocation in Surgery: Bioethics for Clinicians," *Annals RCPSC Supplement* (Fall 1999): 79–81.

the little world around us. Let's try to make whatever difference we can in our surroundings. I believe that this is the only salvation for us. Instead of constantly looking for external help, which is not forthcoming, we need to get up and put our own house in order. If we are not prepared to do this, then we are equally responsible for our quandary. I have conviction that solutions are possible, provided we are all willing to think beyond ourselves. Let us make a difference, one physician at a time.

Eight

HE WHO PAYS THE PIPER CALLS THE TUNE

~

Professional Conduct

Surgery and allied disciplines have made tremendous progress. This has changed the face of surgical practice, all for the good of the patient and the profession. However, I cannot help stating the famous adage that "Everything that is new is not necessarily progress." This cannot be better emphasized than in surgery. Besides the idea that newer is always better, there are many other things that have crept their way into surgical practice: expensive is better, fancier is better, more is better, and so on. One should never be averse to new developments, but there is no reason to indiscriminately latch on to everything that is in vogue.

One needs to remind oneself that the greatest surgical adjunct today is an array of antibiotics available for use in very sick and septic patients. As the organisms are becoming more and more resistant, the newer antibiotics are a blessing when one desperately needs them. A master card must always be used as a last resort. But it is so unfortunate to see the newer generations of antibiotics being abused for simple community-acquired infections. Why would you want to kill a fly with a rocket?

They are expensive and harmful and defy scientific evidence and guidelines. Moreover, very soon, they will suffer the same fate of previous generations. Besides, when the patient really needs these drugs, you will have already used your master card. What are you going to resort to then? First-line drugs?

These practices are so common, especially in places where the practices are largely unregulated. What one forgets is that when one has an outbreak of multidrug-resistant (MDR) organisms or of acinetobacter or candidemia in a hospital, everybody suffers. This is a prime example of collective punishment received because of the irresponsible practices of a few.

Trainees need to reflect on some of these poor practices. They cause immense harm to patients, surgeons, and the health-care system. They are commonly observed when clear guidelines and indications are set aside on personal whims. Where no prophylaxis is indicated, prophylaxis is used; where prophylaxis is indicated, empirical or therapeutic antibiotics are used. Culture sensitivities are treated instead of treating patients, and systemic antibiotics are used instead of local-wound care and drainage. These are the biggest menaces of surgical practice, as one is breeding MDR organisms and superinfections.

The consequences for such irrationality are very high; it leads to significant M&M. MDR sepsis leads to multiorgan dysfunction and failure, requiring critical care and all the related supportive therapy. This makes health care expensive and inaccessible for many. Even with a third-party payer or an insured patient, one must not forget that at the end of the day, the money is coming out of some pocket.

The medical industry has to play a more responsible and mature role and not market newer drugs as if they were distributing candies. Institutions also need to have antibiotic policies and guidelines. Newer generations of antibiotics should be listed as restricted-use drugs. It is a primary obligation of every physician to leave a legacy of good practices. However, it seems that some of us are happy to trade off individual and fleeting successes for long-term, collective punishment and disservice to everybody. However, what we often don't realize is that tomorrow, we will all be in the same soup. It is only a matter of time. The situation requires sensible, rational, and responsible behavior and practices from all stakeholders to stem this catastrophe.

Then one has technology, gadgets, and dubious interventions chasing application. The markets are flooded with all kinds of devices, with newer versions and tall claims of superiority over the previous versions or their competition. They are like cellular phones, which have a new model every six months. Each company has ten different models. Each series has a newer version out before one has even gotten to use the previous one. This is driving the whole world crazy and insulting our intelligence to no end. But who is at fault? The industry or the users? This is true of gadgetry in surgery, too. Unfortunately, the industry here fits hand in glove with the practitioners who are the users. The third party is the unfortunate payer. As long as the practitioners do not have the understanding, confidence, and conviction of what they need and what is available, they can be manipulated by the industry. Patients and health systems will continue to suffer by paying the price. Admittedly, sometimes, there may be marginal benefits, but at what price? Where is the cost-benefit analysis?

We do not have the luxury of unlimited resources, even in the industrialized world. We must be vigilant about reducing health-care costs all around the world. It is morally and ethically incumbent on us to save money, especially in resource-poor settings. However, it is an uphill battle to make surgeons cost-conscious.

The following is a simple example of how the industry can manipulate practitioners. This only happens when one is not sure of what one is doing and what one actually needs to do in a particular job. There are two varieties of colostomy bags. One is an expensive, fancy, two-piece, nontransparent system with a wafer base and a clip-on mechanism. This model has several advantages. It is socially acceptable because the stool is not visible, the wafer base sticks better to skin, and the bags don't have to be changed frequently. When one wishes to empty a bag, one just needs to detach the bag from the ring on the base, empty it, wash it, and clip it back. But it is good for home use and not good for hospital use in the postoperative period.

The other model is a simple, cheap, transparent, disposable bag meant for immediate, postoperative hospital use. Its advantage is that in the postoperative phase, one needs a transparent bag to inspect the stoma for color, bleeding, retraction, edema, and proper functioning. Secondly, the bag needs to be changed more frequently because initially, the content is liquid, large, and unpredictable. Finally, the size of the stoma changes every day due to swelling and edema until it matures. There is no point in providing the patient with an expensive bag that doesn't serve the required medical purpose. However, cheaper and simpler things vanish from the market very quickly, to the extent that people even forget that such a thing ever existed.

When I was annoyed one day with one of the residents because he had opened this fancy, nontransparent, expensive colostomy bag and not the cheap, one-piece, transparent, disposable one, he said, "Which transparent one? I have only seen this one, and everybody uses these bags." This is how the industry pushes us to lose confidence in what we are doing. Instead of need, demand, and reasoning driving the industry, it is the industry driving us to use what they produce. It is so unfortunate, but the industry is winning everywhere.

It is commonly said that the only thing constant in life is change, but change must only come for valid reasons. In the ever-changing world of surgery, you are in a constant state of flux, and the burden of choice is huge. It is our professional responsibility to technically and formally assess the old while concurrently doing the same for the new. Changing without solid reasons reflects poor understanding, lack of self-confidence, and dearth of knowledge. It may even smack of conflict of interest.

Integrity and Conflict of Interest

Medicine is now a thriving industry and a business. There are large profits being made all around. I have lived with guilt all my life for working in a profession where I make my living through human suffering and sickness. But what I see these days pales my guilt. Today, in this industry, patients are called *clients* and doctors are *providers*, a mockery of the sacred, centuries-old patient-doctor relationship. The nexus between the industry and physicians is getting stronger by the hour, and one would be naive to ignore conflicts of interest. Actually, it is no longer a nexus; it is an amorphous cartel that is difficult to discern or detect. There is nothing discreet about it, either. It is now even considered an accepted practice in many places, and medical-council practice guidelines in some countries even allow accruing sponsorships with some caveats, limitations, and declarations of conflict of interest. Is it all so simple?

Today, if we take inventory of the huge and totally unregulated market of implants, equipment, and tools (orthopedic, cardiac, vascular, neurosurgical, interventional, GI, etc.), the claims are tall, and the price differences are huge. I wonder on what basis surgeons decide what is best for their patients.

An industry representative approached me once and offered to fully pay for me to attend an international vascular-surgery conference. I asked him why he was doing me such a big favor. Probably not used to that question, he was a bit surprised, and he mumbled nervously, "Our company believes in supporting continuous professional development, and we are very conscious of our corporate social responsibility . . . blah, blah, blah."

To understand more about this industry benevolence, I asked him, "How else do you support surgeons?" He thought I was now game. He had the courage and audacity to tell me that if I used their vascular grafts, they could negotiate for me to receive a mutually acceptable percentage of the cost of each graft. I immediately asked him, "Are you offering me a kickback?"

Unfortunately, at such times, I can be very rude. I gave him a piece of my mind and his marching orders. But he was not going to go away without having the last word. He apologized to me for insulting my integrity, but he told me that it was uncommon. He said that his agency was the sole local distributor for many orthopedic and vascular implants and many supplies and disposables. Then he threw on the table some visiting cards of the leading surgeons with whom they had negotiated deals. He told me that the practice was so rampant and open that it was accepted as a norm and that by refusing such an offer, I was being a loser. I hung my head in shame and had nothing more to say. After that, whenever I saw appliances and implants from that supplier being religiously used by some, I felt sick to my stomach.

One morning, I walked into the surgeons' room in the operating rooms. One of our former orthopedic trainees, who is now a busy consultant orthopedic surgeon in another city, was sitting there. He jumped up from his seat as soon as he saw me and greeted me very fondly and with great respect. We sat down and started chatting about almost everything.

Somewhere along the discussion, I asked him, "What orthopedic implants do you use in your practice?" He mentioned a particularly renowned manufacturing company. I asked him if there was any particular reason for this choice. He said that he was trained in a center where they commonly used these implants and equipment. I asked him if he exclusively used their products. He said yes. I then pointed out that there are so many other good companies around and that they may even have better implants, which may be even cheaper.

"Have you tried them?" I asked. He said that he had a good relationship with this manufacturer and that they provided him with excellent service and equipment. Upon further probing, he said they also funded him every year for his professional development and funded a visit of one of his mentors for a week to his place to do some complex work. I felt too embarrassed and ashamed to explore any further the depth of this relationship. It left me wondering about this strange phenomenon where one has great reverence for a former teacher but not much respect for his teachings. I would have been much happier if things had been other way around. Unfortunately, that is not often the case.

Without the industry, medicine would have not made as much progress. But today, the industry is big, powerful, and making huge profits. They are throwing some crumbs at physicians in the name of research funding, continuous professional development, and support of scientific conferences and workshops. Unfortunately, there is no dearth of takers; on the contrary, there is a scramble for such support in some parts of the world. The amount and level of support accorded depends on how big and influential one is as an organization or as an individual. Some of the trainees are also not behind in claiming their share of the pie, but what they get at the end of the day defies any logic or reason. We have sold ourselves for a pot of puree.[24]

It is not about the price, though; it's about the principle. What we mustn't forget is that there are no free lunches anywhere; as the adage states, "He who pays the piper calls the tune." Not surprisingly, today, we must teach trainees to understand conflict of interest and combat this onslaught on our professional values and integrity. In my experience, the simple policy of declaring conflicts of interest has made no difference. There must be stricter regulation and oversight surrounding the physician-industry nexus. It is also important for us to reflect individually on our relationship with the industry in light of our own moral underpinnings.

Lesson on Life

On my return from the West, I was not very busy, and I decided to dedicate some of my time to a charitable hospital. I found one right downtown in a very poor and densely populated area where many people would not even like to venture. I just wanted to be accessible to poor people by rendering my free services. I felt that it was my payback time.

One day, I finished a long operating list in the afternoon, and I walked to the changing room while chatting with the senior male OR tech. Engrossed in the chat, I removed the scrub-suit top. It had my wristwatch in the top pocket, and the watch came out and smashed on the opposite wall and fell on the floor. The tech immediately picked it up, and after seeing it, he said he was sorry that the second hand had come out and was lying on the dial. He told me that just behind the hospital, there was a guy with a small roadside cart who repaired watches. The tech told me that I should just go to him and that he would fix it. I told him not to worry because it was a cheap, fake watch, which just looked good and genuine. I thanked him anyway, and I said that I would think about getting it fixed.

---

24 Augusto Sarmiento, "Medicine and Industry: The Payer, the Piper and the Tune," *Annals CRMCC* 23, no. 3 (2000): 144–149.

I finished my post-op round, and as I walked down the stairs and through the crowded corridors full of poor patients, I changed my mind. I decided to venture out to the back street of the hospital just for kicks.

There was a long, narrow, dusty alley next to the hospital, which led me to a small, quiet street at the rear of the hospital. I looked around, and on my right some meters away, there was a small two-by-two-by-four-foot wooden cart on four small wheels parked on the footpath. There was guy sitting on a high stool under a small, torn, tattered canopy to avoid the sun. He had a small glass cabin over this cart, and inside it, he displayed old, antique table clocks and wristwatches and a half-open drawer below, in which he had his tools.

He was a very pleasant middle-aged man with a broad smile on his face. He welcomed me and was clearly surprised. Based on my attire, he knew that I did not fit the profile of his local customers. After an exchange of pleasantries, he gave me another stool to sit on next to him under his shade. I gave him my wristwatch, and he looked at it and said, "No problem. I will fix it in two minutes." In the meantime, he shouted across the street to a small tea shop and ordered two cups of tea. Within no time, a boy brought a small rusted steel teapot with two small ceramic teacups with no handles or saucers. The boy poured the tea, and with a cool breeze blowing, a young surgeon and a seasoned watchmaker sipped nice, strong, hot tea as they sat on the roadside.

As we talked, he quickly put on his magnifying eyepiece and opened the back cover of the wristwatch. He then turned it around and gently tapped it on his palm, and the watch machinery came out of the casing. He softly brushed the dial and put a little superglue on the center pin of the dial and pressed the second hand back on the pin. He reversed the exercise in the same order and tightened back the lid. He adjusted the time, cleaned the watch, and handed it over to me. "It will never come out again," he said.

I thanked him for the nice cup of tea and asked him the price for his service. He first said, "Nothing." When I asked why, he said, "Because you are a guest." When I insisted on paying, he said, "One rupee" (less than one cent). This is when he very well knew that I could afford to pay him any decent amount.

I stood up and said, "You must be joking." He said he had never charged anybody more than five rupees for his labor. This was no job. I told him, "You gave me a cup of tea and did a job for which you do not wish to charge. How do you survive?"

He said, "Would you charge a guest for a cup of tea you serve him?" He pointed to the opposite ancient and derelict building and said that he lived there in a small one-bedroom apartment with his wife. He earned enough to respectfully sustain the two of them. After sunset, he would push his cart under the staircase at the entrance of his building and go up to his apartment. According to him, the poor people of this locality gave him work; he charged them whatever they could pay, and it was enough for his sustenance.

"Why do I need more money? I am happy. My needs are being fulfilled, and I sleep well and peacefully at night," he said with a smile of serenity. I was just speechless, listening to his philosophy and seeing the level of deep contentment and happiness. I tried to give him one hundred rupees, and he said, "Now you are trying to help me, and I don't need any help. I am not poor." He finally and reluctantly took five rupees.

I was so glad that I had made that small detour; otherwise, I would have never received such a beautiful lesson on life. To some, the watch mender may appear to be a pauper sitting on the roadside, but he left me in pure awe. He seemed to me the proudest, richest, happiest, most dignified, and most contented soul on Earth.

We have unfortunately all fallen into the rat race and the rut of chasing—rightfully or wrongfully—what is and isn't our due. Despite amassing so much, if we truly look within ourselves, we are genuinely poor on all accounts. We have forgotten that no amount of material gain can buy us intrinsic happiness and contentment. How fortunate we are to be in a profession where we have an immense opportunity to gain true, eternal happiness and contentment every day. Moreover, this will surely help us to sleep well and peacefully at night, too—something worth thinking about.

Nine

By Failing to Prepare, You Are Preparing to Fail

~

By failing to prepare, you are preparing to fail.

—Benjamin Franklin

Surgical Blues

Surgical blues are cases, events, and happenings in one's surgical career that come under the umbrella of medical errors. We all know that patient safety today is a major agenda of health care around the world. Diagnostic errors, poor judgment, communication breakdowns, and inadequate skills can directly result in patient harm and even death. I will narrate a few classical cases here that epitomize all the discussed causes of medical error. There was a lot of learning from these cases for our team, the institution, and myself. These cases still haunt me; they make me sad, depressed, and even despairing. If you are willing, there is a lot to learn from these stories for everybody who is aspiring to be a surgeon or is in the business of patient care.

Chronology of Disasters

One night in the '90s, a twenty-one-year-old was brought to our emergency department after sustaining a road-traffic accident. He was sitting in a coaster bus on the front seat alongside the driver when it rammed into the back of a static large articulated truck. It was nighttime; the road was unlit, and the driver missed it completely. The driver died on the spot, and he was extricated and evacuated.

On arrival, the patient was hemodynamically unstable with polytrauma, so a trauma call was activated. The trauma team managed him well, according to the advance-trauma life-support (ATLS) protocol then. The patient had lateral cervical spine (C-spine), chest, and pelvic X-rays, which were all cleared as normal by the trauma team and the radiology senior resident on call. Both the patient's lower limbs were mangled due to crushing injury. His Glasgow Coma Scale (GCS) was 15/15, and his breathing was spontaneous. The patient stabilized after resuscitation. His abdomen was passed as benign. His cervical collar was removed, and the patient was handed over to the orthopedic team for further care and management.

They took him to the operating room that same night and did an above-knee amputation on the left side. The right also required an above-knee amputation. Because it was slightly better than the left and the patient was very young, they decided to do an extensive debridement in this sitting. The patient had two more visits to the operating room over the following five days for rechecks and debridement. In all, he had a total of three general anesthetics (GAs) administered to him with intubation and ventilation. Given his severe bilateral lower-limb and soft-tissue injuries, the nurses were regularly turning him in his bed to prevent pressure sores.

On day five in the HDU, the nurses in their usual style held the bedsheet under the patient and pulled to turn the patient. One, two, three—*zip*—the patient was turned with a jerk, and he was rendered quadriplegic. They immediately called the surgical team, and neurosurgery came on board. They reviewed the ER lateral C-spine X-ray. This was reported the next morning by the consultant radiologist, who raised radiological suspicion of a C4 over C5 (cervical vertebrae) slip and possible instability. A clinical correlation was recommended, and a CAT scan was advised. The report was filed, and nobody ever saw it once the patient was handed over to the orthopods. The patient had had three GAs and intubations, and nothing had happened until this episode.

The nurse who had been looking after him during the day for the last four days was very distraught. She came forward and volunteered that during these days, the mother had been doing oil massages of the patient's head. Every time she did the head massage, the patient would complain of tingling in both arms. When the mother informed the nurse, she stopped the mother from doing the massage. She was devastated that she could not put two plus two together. She was distraught, thinking that she could have at least reported it to the team, even though she herself had not understood the warning signs. How much I admire her for her honesty and profound feeling of regret.

The neurosurgeons in those days were in the practice of using immediate and very heavy doses of methylprednisolone in acute spinal-cord injuries. I am not sure what they believe today, as this wheel has turned so many times that I have lost track of it. The neurosurgeons have been flirting with steroids from time immemorial, but they have never solemnized this affair. I am not sure if they ever will, at least not in my lifetime. The patient was hit with heavy doses of steroids. A CAT scan revealed unstable anterior subluxation of C4 over C5. They took him to the operating room and did a cervical fusion of the unstable level.

Now we had a twenty-one-year-old patient with crushed and amputated lower limbs who was quadriplegic. Neurosurgery and orthopedics were on board now, but neurosurgery was the driver, and orthopedics had taken a back seat. Eight days after this event, our chief resident in general surgery was doing his evening exit round on HDU. He was asked by a first-year neurosurgery resident to assist him in passing the NGT. He was having difficulty passing it. He asked the story of the patient and the reason that he was passing an NGT. The unfortunate disaster was narrated to him. He was also told that in the last two days, the patient had developed abdominal distension, and this was thought to be meteorism. An NGT was being passed to decompress the bowel.

It was great that our chief resident did not buy the diagnosis and decided to examine the patient's abdomen. It was insensate; the patient was not complaining of pain and no tenderness could be elicited. He could only detect distension. However, the resident very cleverly observed that the patient had loss of liver dullness on percussion. Given that the patient was on heavy doses of steroids and due to the risk of stress ulceration, he suspected a perforated DU. He asked for a portable, supine, decubitus X-ray of the abdomen. Sure enough, it showed pneumoperitoneum.

Now general surgeons were on board, too, and the other two specialties took a back seat. I was informed, and although it was evening, I was still in my office. After resuscitation, the patient was taken to the operating room. I remember I was at the red line in the operating room. The chief resident said he was happy and confident dealing with it. He asked me to sit in my office and said that he would call me if needed. He found an at-least-two-day-old perforation (if not more), and things were quite friable. He patched the perforation, did a copious washout, and left a big drain along the subhepatic area and closed the abdomen.

The patient was now septic; he was ventilated and shifted to the ICU. He was already going through a stormy postoperative course when, on the third day, the drain started leaking bile. The closure had broken down. He developed a high-output fistula—yet another catastrophe. In the next few days, he continued to show signs of sepsis. A CAT scan showed interloop abscesses and collections not amenable to image-guided drainage.

We decided to go in to deal with the abscesses, do a good washout, establish good external drainage, and pass the NGT across the fistula for continuous suction to reduce output. TPN was very expensive, and with its septic and metabolic complications, we were inclined to establish an enteral route via a feeding jejunostomy. We did all that during the second laparotomy. The bowel was edematous, and we did not close the abdomen due to fear of compartment syndrome. We left the abdomen open and stitched around a Vicryl mesh to the sheath edges for covering the bowel loops and for dressing.

The patient did well for a week when he suddenly developed a brisk hemorrhage from the upper end of the wound through the mesh. This was enough to make him hemodynamically unstable, and we had to go in again to explore. Everything was edematous, friable, and plastered. We just followed the tract of the hemorrhage. At every step, we felt as if we were going to make a hole in the bowel. We were lucky; with a lot of irrigation fluid and delicate maneuvers, we were able to gingerly separate the bowel loops. We finally reached the infracolic compartment, where a small abscess had eroded into the middle colic vessels. We ligated them and closed in the same fashion as before.

The patient again slowly stabilized, and then ten days later, he developed a small-bowel fistula from the lower end of the wound. I think a small abscess eroded into the bowel, and the fistula was now distal to the feeding jejunostomy—yet another disaster. It had been way over a month now, and we had had one catastrophe after the other.

We now had a twenty-one-year-old patient who was mentally alert with a tracheostomy and who was ventilated with minimal support, growing nasty MDR acinetobacter from the trachea, and quadriplegic with an amputated left leg, a crushed and functionally useless right leg, multiple entercutaneous fistulas, and sepsis. Even if he came out of all this, what kind of quality of life would he have in the context of a developing country?

The team had no conviction that we should go any further. The patient and his mother wanted him to live, even as a disabled person. I still remember the patient asking me once, "Will I be all right? I want to live and go home." We kept giving him hope. Yet we neither had hope nor any conviction in what we were doing. We continued to do whatever was possible. He eventually succumbed after two months and eleven days.

It may have been a blessing in disguise for him. But we, the living ones, were left with events to haunt us forever: the trauma team who passed the lateral C-spine as normal; the radiologists who suspected something and did not alert the primary team; the residents and consultants who did not validate their X-ray findings of the night with radiologists the next day; the nurse who was informed of tingling of arms secondary to vigorous head movement and could not understand the meaning; the use of heavy doses of steroids; ulcer prophylaxis; and not being alert to the complications, especially in an insensate abdomen. Should I have scrubbed for the case to repair a perforated DU, and would it have made a difference? The rest is all history.

We all had lots of emotional baggage and guilt, and it was not easy for anybody. But besides feeling profound regret, we could not do anything. However, we promptly changed our systems, and a lot of processes were improved as we learned from every step of this case, which I refer to as a *chronology of disasters.*

Fatal Error

Nights are synonymous with darkness and evil, and there is nothing good written about them in folklore. Hospitals are no different; the majority of the catastrophes happen during the darkness of night. I still teach residents that if you can do something in broad daylight, don't do it at night. Don't make any major decisions about removing tubes, drains, a bedside procedure, or shifting a patient at night.

Nighttime is for doing what is absolutely essential. Don't write PRN/ SOS (Latin *pro re nata*, meaning "save our souls"—as and when required) analgesia because it often gets administered at night so that the nurse and the patient can sleep peacefully. Don't send an inpatient down for an X-ray that could not be done during the day. Always follow the verbal reports or even written reports given during the night; they frequently get changed completely in the morning.

I have frequently wondered why this is the case. It is multifactorial. Many of the reasons are genuine, such as overworked and skeleton staff during odd hours. Some are purely due to professionalism and attitude. There is a term and position in cricket called the *night watchman.* He is the worst of the batters, and he's sent only to bat and hold the fort for the night. Nobody expects him to start hitting boundaries or dispatch the ball out of the park. The next morning, he gets clean bowled on the first ball. But that is fine as he has done the job he was assigned to do. I have learned to look at some of the staff on night duty in hospitals as night watchmen. I try to put in all my precautionary measures, and then I am less worried about what happens at night in my absence.

Once in the middle of the night, we were doing an emergency surgery. The chief resident and a second-year resident were with me, and the team was called for urgent help for my twenty-three-year-old, postlaparotomy, polytrauma patient who was in the ICU. Two days previously, he had been in a road-traffic accident and sustained a head injury, a left chest injury with rib fractures, and a ruptured spleen. He had a left chest tube inserted for pneumohemothorax and a laparotomy for trauma splenectomy. He was being ventilated because of his low GCS, but otherwise, he was stable. The ICU nurse informed that the patient had suddenly started to desaturate and had become tachycardic and hypotensive. They had challenged him with fluid boluses, but he was not responding.

We were finishing, and I left the residents to close and went to see the patient. When I arrived at the ICU, the patient was having CPR. While standing at the foot of the bed and wondering what had happened, I noticed that the chest tube had a Spencer Wells forceps clamped on it. I leapt forward and took off the clamp, and I have never seen so much bubbling ever in the underwater seal bottle. A pool nurse had emptied the underwater-seal bottle, and after reattaching it, she had forgotten to remove the clamp. The CPR was unsuccessful, and the patient died of tension pneumothorax on an ICU.

I looked at the data on the monitor; the sudden dip in the vitals had occurred half an hour ago, and it corroborated with the event. It was a classical picture of tension pneumothorax. The irony was that there was a clear and substantive rise in airway pressure, and even the machine was buzzing the alarm. This was silenced because it was thought to be erroneous. Ironically, they increased the positive end expiratory pressure (PEEP) to maximum in order to improve saturations! There was a locum medical officer in the ICU who had the blank look of a night watchman. Sometimes, I wonder whether we need bodies to hold the fort or people with some competence. Mere bodies give one a sense of illusory comfort. Unfortunately, their incompetence is a source of much greater harm.

Crucial Miss

A couple was involved in a road-traffic accident on a single highway. Both were restrained passengers, and in avoiding an oncoming vehicle, they went off the road and flipped their car. It was two in the morning on an intercity road. They were extricated from the vehicle and taken to a nearby small hospital. They received resuscitation and were transferred to our facility, arriving at around six in the morning.

The husband, fifty-eight years old, was relatively stable, conscious, alert, and sitting up on the couch. He had a left chest tube, which was swinging with blood-tinged fluid in the bottle. The chief resident stated that the patient was fine, and it was his fifty-two-year-old wife who was pale and unstable. She had responded to the bolus, and they had done a CAT scan. She had a grade II liver laceration and a grade IV splenic injury with free fluid. She also had an acute ischemia of the left lower limb due to direct blunt trauma to the groin, resulting in thrombosis of the femoral artery. The husband kept telling us to see his wife because he was fine.

We took the lady to the operating room and did a splenectomy. While we were doing the femoral embolectomy on her, we were informed that the husband has suddenly poured two liters of frank blood from his chest tube and arrested. CPR was being done.

He was revived and was immediately wheeled into the operating room, and we did a quick left thoracotomy. The chest was full of blood, and he arrested again as we entered. We started an open cardiac massage, but the heart was empty; he had exsanguinated. He could not be revived. The mediastinum around the mid–thoracic aorta was wide, with a contained hematoma. This had ruptured at one point, creating a large buttonhole. When I opened the mediastinal pleura and removed the clot, I found the descending thoracic aorta inside completely transected. Looking back at the chest X-ray from the peripheral hospital, one could see a subtle widening of the mediastinum in the region. He had remained relatively stable for six hours until our resuscitation popped the hematoma.

Trauma is so deceptive and complex. Things get even more complicated when patients are transferred from another facility. Already, some halfhearted interventions have been done, and some time has been lost. One also erroneously starts thinking that the time lapse itself is suggestive of hemodynamic stability and lack of any major injury. Always be aware of the ones who look well, and never shortchange your assessment based on deceptive external appearances. Approach every trauma patient and every transfer from other facilities as if you are the first medical help to the patient; you will never regret it.

Friday-Afternoon Syndrome

Friday afternoon is a bad time anywhere to get anybody's time or attention. This is true of hospitals as well. This is when many omissions and blunders happen. Unfortunately, the price of this is too high in our profession.

We once did a femoropopliteal bypass on a seventy-two-year-old gentleman with a reversed long-saphenous-vein graft. I was a surgical registrar then on the vascular unit. On Wednesday, the fifth post-op day, the upper end of the wound was showing signs of infection. I removed three stitches, let the pus out, and sent it for culture and sensitivity. Empirical antibiotics were started. The patient was otherwise well and ambulant. I held his discharge to see how the wound would respond. I was worried about a secondary hemorrhage.

On Friday, I looked at the wound; it appeared slightly worse. I chased the culture-sensitivity report. They said it would be out by the afternoon. I put it out of my mind. I was off that weekend and traveled somewhere.

On Monday morning, I found that at three on Saturday morning, the patient had been found dead in his bed. The bed and floor were covered with blood. He had bled to death in his sleep. The practice on the surgical floors is that the patients who are well and near discharge are shifted to bays at the end of the ward. Acute patients are kept in closer bays near the nursing stations. He was unfortunately in the last bay.

I quickly checked his culture-sensitivity report. It showed nasty gram-negative bugs, which were not sensitive to the antibiotics I was giving. The postmortem revealed death due to an exsanguinating secondary hemorrhage from an almost-complete disruption of saphenofemoral anastomosis. Whether it would have made a difference or not to the outcome, the moral burden of such costly omissions remains with you forever.

There is no issue if you are scheduled to be off work; everybody is entitled to some time off. However, since this incident, all my life, I have been paranoid about proper handing over of my patients while I'm going away, especially those I am particularly concerned about. Teams must have proper and appropriate handing over and taking over (documented) at both exit and entry rounds. Many types of software are available on smartphones to facilitate this, and all resident and training programs must use them. Even faculty can receive information on their phones about the handing-over information of their patients.

Near Miss

Most often, I do my daily exit round alone. This helps me assess resident teams' thinking and management plans and review their documentation. It also gives me an opportunity to see relatives, who are mostly there at that time.

One evening, I was rounding on my patient in HDU. I was focused on the patient, his parameters, and charting. I heard the nurse telling the senior student nurse to connect the feed and that she was just coming. When she left, the student nurse attached the drip set to the commercially prepared five-hundred-milliliter packet of enteral feed. She let the air out and connected it. I was watching, but my mind was focused more on the patient. I stayed for a while, looked at the notes, talked to the patient, and then left.

As I walked out of the ward and was going down the stairs, it occurred to me to check whether the enteral feed was connected to the central line or the nasojejunal tube. I thought I had seen something odd, but it had not registered in my mind. I decided to go back and check. Sure enough, it was connected to the central line. Luckily, only a small amount had gone in, and nothing much happened to the patient. It is so easy to make mistakes.

Managing the Monster

Makary and Daniel report in a recently published study that if medical error were a disease, it would be reported as the third-leading cause of death in the United States.[25] And these are just indirect estimates and extrapolations. We all know that nobody has ever listed a cause of death as a *medical error*. There is underreporting, too, due to fear of retribution and medicolegal implications for the individual and the institution. If there were real estimates, medical error would surely be the number-one cause of death.

The same study proposes a three-tiered approach to error management. First, the error should be made visible. We must create a culture of reporting errors. Second, we must respond to the error. And third, we must make errors less frequent by taking preventive measures and improving systems and processes.

Lucian Leape, a Harvard pediatrician who is also referred to as the father of patient safety, first drew the analogy in his special communication in the *Journal of the American Medical Association* (*JAMA*) in 1994 that the number of deaths due to medical error in the United States is equivalent to three jumbo jets crashing every other day.[26] The figures are much higher now. A World Health Organization (WHO) report states that health care has a poorer safety record than any other high-risk industry. There is a one-in-a-million chance of a traveler being harmed while in an aircraft. In comparison, there is a

---

25 Martin Makary and Michael Daniel, "Medical Error—The Third Leading Cause of Death in the US," *British Medical Journal* 353 (2016): i2139.

26 Lucian Leape, "Error in Medicine," *JAMA* 272, no. 23 (December 21, 1994): 1851–1857.

one-in-three-hundred chance of a patient being harmed during health care.[27]

An estimated 234 million surgical operations are performed globally every year.[28] Surgical procedures carry a significant burden of errors; almost 50 percent of complications associated with surgical care are avoidable. The delivery of safe surgery requires a team approach. Safety studies have shown that additional hospitalization, litigation costs, infections acquired in hospitals, disability, lost productivity, and medical expenses cost some countries as much as US$19 billion annually. About 20 percent to 40 percent of all health spending is wasted due to poor-quality care. The economic benefits of improving patient safety are therefore compelling.

There is now growing recognition that patient safety and quality is a universal, critical dimension of health care. It is unacceptable that anybody should be allowed to fall victim to a human or system error or an act of omission. Adverse events may result from problems in practice, products, procedures, or systems. Patient-safety improvements demand a complex, system-wide effort involving a wide range of actions in performance improvement, environmental safety, risk management, infection control, safe use of medicines, equipment safety, and safe clinical practice.

WHO's patient-safety curriculum for medical schools must be integrated into medical education.[29] It is high time that medical error be classified as an endemic disease prevalent worldwide and acknowledged openly. The textbooks should include chapters on and time allocated for formal education, sensitization, and awareness of patient-safety issues. Implementing and meeting standards of WHO patient-surgical-safety checklists and the national and international patient-safety goals (IPSGs)

---

27 "Ten Facts on Patient Safety," World Health Organization, http://www.who.int/features/factfiles/patient_safety/patient_safety_facts/en/index6.html.

28 "WHO Guidelines on Patient Safety," World Health Organization, http://www.who.int/publications/guidelines/patient_safety/en/.

29 "Patient Safety," World Health Organization, http://www.who.int/patientsafety/education/curriculum/download/en/.

of the Joint Commission International (JCI) are important benchmarks to achieve in error management.[30]

All this looks and sounds good as we learn many lessons from the airline industry. There are surely a lot of low-hanging fruits. We can improve our safety standards by taking simple measures to avoid errors and by implementing patient-safety goals. However, the practice of medicine unfortunately cannot be realistically equated to or compared with the airline industry. There are many confounding variables introduced by the human element (caregivers and patients), which are unpredictable and difficult to influence.

Two patients with the same diagnosis are never the same. No two surgeons think or act alike. A human being is not a jumbo jet or an Airbus. After following checklists, algorithms, protocols, and pathways to their limit and with all the time-outs and sign-outs, we eventually enter the realms of human elements: physician reaction and the patient response. This is not a science per se; it is not reproducible and cannot be predictable or prescriptive. The checklists are surely essential to preventing acts of omission or oversight or system errors, as we have learned from the airline industry. However, it would be naive to ignore the differences. Recognition of these specific challenges would help the larger error-management issues.

---

30 For further information, see Ed Kelley, "An Overview of WHO Patient Safety: An Opportunity for New Collaboration," World Health Organization, February 2, 2010, http://ec.europa.eu/health/patient_safety/docs/ev_20100202 _co03_en.pdf; "National Patient Safety Goals," The Joint Commission, https:// www.jointcommission.org/standards_information/npsgs.aspx; and "International Patient Safety Goals," Joint Commission International, http://www. jointcommissioninternational.org/improve/international-patient-safety-goals.

Ten

A Turtle Makes Progress When It Sticks Its Neck Out

—

A turtle makes progress when it sticks its neck out.

—James Bryant Conant

The Buck Stops Here

In surgery, decision-making is the toughest thing. Inability to make tough decisions and passing the buck to others does not help anybody; it unfortunately just becomes a merry-go-round for the poor patients.

Sometimes, you find nothing wrong with the patients, but you are hesitant to tell patients that there is nothing wrong with them. Ideally, you should explain unambiguously and convincingly to the patients that there is nothing wrong with them. Give them a clean bill of health. Who would not be happy to hear the news that all is well unless someone is a hypochondriac?

Instead, there is a common tendency to hand over some analgesic prescription, gel, cream, unnecessary test, referral, or repeat appointment. This way, you are acknowledging that there is something wrong with the patient. Also, one gives them hope that whatever is wrong with them will get better with the medicine or will be sorted out by someone else. Previously, the patients only thought that there was something wrong with them. Now the patients believe that even the doctor thinks that there is something wrong, but as the doctor doesn't understand the problem, they need to go to someone else. This is how the vicious cycle starts when it should have been ended at the first consult.

It is particularly sad when these decisions are about life and death. It is understandable for the patient to be in denial, but how can a surgeon be in denial? By sending the patient to someone else, the surgeon gives the patient hope. Unfortunately, by doing so, we also take away from patients the hope of dying a good death. Do not promise what others cannot deliver.

We all know and understand that hope is a necessary part of the will to live and fight disease. But why do we forget that we are all mere mortals and perishable souls? Why is it that when death is staring into the eyes of the patients, each one of us is passing the buck to somebody else? This prolongs their misery and suffering by dubious and unnecessary surgical interventions or by some highly poisonous and toxic palliative or rescue chemotherapy, all with marginal benefits.

The unfortunate part is that we all feel when we receive a patient that we must do something, all in good faith. But somebody somewhere must stop and ask, what we are doing and achieving here? I know this is the most difficult part, and hence, everybody keeps postponing it until it's too late. We must realize that when we avoid discussing the reality of dying with our patients, we are causing more harm by perpetuating and inflicting a lot of human, spiritual, social, and economic suffering. The basic premise is that the buck stops with you as the surgeon. You will have to make these bold decisions; no one else will make them.

On January 1, 2000, the first day of the new millennium, I had to operate on an unfortunate thirty-two-year-old male for a poorly differentiated signet-ring-cell type of adenocarcinoma of the stomach. Given that he was a young patient with a bad type of tumor biology, I did a D2 radical gastrectomy. He received full adjuvant therapy and spent the rest of the first nine months after the diagnosis in and out of the hospital.

Tumor biology is king.[31] Just as the patient was now returning back to normal life with a hope of being cured, he presented with a small-bowel obstruction nine months after finishing his treatment. Recurrence of the disease was likely. But a CAT scan did not detect any gross disease, and there was an abrupt cutoff in the small bowel. Exploration revealed peritoneal disease, and we did an internal bypass to relieve his obstruction. In the tumor board, there was talk of second-line palliative chemotherapy.

I sat with the patient and his young wife and told them in so many words that there was no hope for a cure now. We could not cure him, but we would surely take care of him. We would help him and support him all the way with pain management, nutritional therapy, and any other palliative care. They were devastated. I told them that the option of palliative chemotherapy was always there and to let me know if they decided to exercise that option, and we would organize it.

One month later, the patient came to my clinic with his wife and his two beautiful kids just to say thank you. He was thankful to me for putting him out of this misery and false hope. He said, "It was not easy at first. But by letting me know that my time is up, you gave me the opportunity to do so many things. Many people do not get to do that. I enjoy my time with the kids. I have gone out and visited so many people I had not seen in years. I have said sorry to people I needed to. I do things that I always wanted to do. I eat what I want to eat. I have sorted out my accounts and my property. Above all, I look at everything in the world as if I will not see it again. Suddenly, everything around me seems so beautiful. I am at peace with myself, and I am enjoying every second I have left of my life." He stood up, very warmly shook hands with me, and left with a broad smile on his face.

---

31 Blake Cady, "Principles in Surgical Oncology," *Archives of Surgery* 132(4) (April 1997): 338–346.

The next time I saw him was when he was admitted under me as an emergency due to vomiting induced by a cocktail of narcotics and advancing disease. He was severely emaciated, dehydrated, and drowsy but still compos mentis. He said, "Doc, my time is up; just keep me comfortable." He died very peacefully two days later with all his family around, twenty-two months after the diagnosis.

On another occasion, I was called early in the morning by a colleague physician consultant to see one of his patients. The ninety-year-old lady had some vague abdominal pains and mild distension but no other signs. I asked him if she was constipated. He very unconvincingly said that he did not think so. I know physicians would rather do a CAT scan or a colonoscopy than do a rectal examination. It drives me crazy when they send a consult for acute abdomen for a patient who turns out to be constipated. I asked him if there was any urgency; he said not at all. I told him I would pass by.

I walked across the hospital to their ward at around eleven in the morning. The sister on the ward told me the bed number and name of the patient and said she would join me shortly, as she was talking to a relative. I approached this patient, and she seemed to be sleeping. Then I realized that she was not breathing. I checked her pulse and then the heartbeat, and it seemed she had passed away without anybody realizing. I put her straight and covered her up and walked back. As I reached the sister's office, I bumped into the consultant and told him that she passed away very peacefully without the help of yet another doctor.

Sometimes, recognition of the phenomena of dying in such situations would help patients die peacefully and reduce the misery of their families. It would also save other colleagues from unnecessary referrals and the burden of decision-making.

I have had the privilege of seeing a lot of compassion, greatness, and resilience in patients' families. Much of the suffering one sees is unnecessary and avoidable. It comes about when we as caregivers hide behind our fear of death and postpone dealing with the reality of dying until it is too late. This is all because we are all prepared and programmed during our training to work at the goal of preserving life. What we forget is that we can switch goals to reduce human suffering and move to the goal of providing a good, dignified death. There is nothing wrong or unethical about it. After all, we all have to die of something someday. I believe there is dignity of the living and dignity of the dying, and everybody is entitled to a dignified death; we need to respect this.

Captain of the Ship

In maritime law, the captain of the ship is held liable for the negligence of members of his or her crew. This analogy of *captain of the ship* was first applied to medical malpractice in the case of *McConnell v. Williams* (1949) in the United States.[32] The referenced article is a very interesting read about the evolution of this analogy and the way that it has been historically applied to only medical malpractice cases. The captain-of-the-ship legacy holds surgeons liable for the actions of everyone in operating rooms, whether one controls their actions or not. According to this article, "The problem has been the surgeons who have liked and identified with the romantic notion of being 'captain of the ship' and were unwilling to admit that there were activities in the operating room which they did not control."[33] The defendant lawyers have regularly challenged the courts, and there is an understanding that it is not one's assumption of the role but one's ability to control things that matters.

In surgery, there are independent, certified, and credentialed care providers who partner with us and work in operating rooms all the time to anesthetize patients. During the period that the patient is asleep, they monitor and manage the patient's respiratory, cardiac, hemodynamic, cerebral, metabolic, and renal physiology while the surgeons are busy and engrossed in their handicraft with all kinds of anatomical and nonanatomical resections, repairs, reconstructions, fixations, explants, implants, and transplants.

---

32 Gene Blumenreich, "Captain of the Ship," *Journal of American Nurse Anesthetists* 61, no. 1 (February 1991): 3–6.

33 Ibid., 4.

The surgeon remains the team leader, but this relationship has to be complementary and professional. It must be based on mutual respect and understanding of roles and responsibilities. The anesthetist must be competent and prepared to handle all the stresses and strains being put on the body by surgical trauma. The surgeon should be competent and proficient enough to deal with the problems efficiently and without major and abrupt challenges to patient physiology, such as a hemorrhage. If there is an anticipated step that is likely to produce instability or unexpected hemorrhage, it is better to warn the anesthetist rather than allow him or her to be informed by abrupt fluctuations of vitals, sudden commotion, or the sucker bottle filling up. Also, the surgeon should be prepared to temporarily stop while the patient is being stabilized, to abbreviate the procedure, or even to wind up and call it a day if the anesthetist believes that proceeding further would jeopardize the life of the patient. Although there are individual roles, responsibilities, and accountabilities, there is also shared liability.

A long time ago, when I had recently returned from England, I operated on four patients and removed retained swabs from previous operations. One eighteen-year-old patient died, and three others suffered significant morbidity. Three patients had small four-by-four swabs, and one had a large abdominal pack left after a C-section. I thought that if I, one surgeon, had removed four swabs in six months, there must be many other patients being operated on by others elsewhere with a similar problem. I decided to present all four cases in the citywide, monthly Society of Surgeons meeting.

On the day of my presentation, the hall was full of surgeons, and I presented briefly the story of all four cases, all anonymously and without reference to any surgeon or hospital. I also admitted that due to cost constraints, Raytec swabs were not available in many hospitals, which was part of the problem. At the end of the presentation, I posed some questions: Even if one uses Raytec swabs, they still must be accounted for at the end of an operation, so why was there no reliable swab count done? Who was ultimately responsible for this debacle? Finally, what systems and processes can we put in place to ensure that this doesn't happen again?

Initially, there was silence. Then there was at least acceptance and acknowledgment that it was a major problem. But when it came time to assigning responsibility, there was pandemonium. Some felt that the surgeon was the captain of the ship. Others felt that the hospital, the staff, and the scrub nurses were responsible for it. Some even said that the staff were very ill trained, unprofessional, and untrustworthy. There were others who said that they worked in a very difficult environment and were already stressed out with so many other things on their mind. Therefore, the accountability for the swabs could not be put in the surgeon's lap.

It was all unbelievable and sad. Eventually, I said what I felt. No matter what, it is ultimately the surgeon's responsibility to ensure that there is credible accounting for swabs, needles, and instruments at the end of the procedure. Failure to do this results in patient M&M. Moreover, as captain of the ship, this is one domain that is under the surgeon's control, so we cannot absolve ourselves of this responsibility.

I suggested that we should stop using small swabs in deep cavities unless they were on an instrument. Otherwise, they were more likely to be lost or forgotten. If one did decide to use them, then make sure everybody was alerted to remind them to remove the swab and ensure a reliable swab count was taken at the end of the procedure. Surgeons cannot abdicate this responsibility to anybody else. Ultimately, the patient is the surgeon's ethical, moral, and professional responsibility, and the surgeon will also be held liable for not ensuring a credible system as a team leader in operating rooms.

Therefore, as a matter of law, surgeons are assumed to be in control of the personnel in operating rooms, and they are liable as the captain of the ship for negligence. However, surgeons are normally not in full control of all personnel in operating rooms. This is clear in the two scenarios I have narrated above. Despite this, surgeons could be indirectly held responsible for their role in negligence, such as for the choice of a competent anesthetist, support provided to the team as a leader, recognition of instability of the patient, the role as a surgeon in creating that instability, assistance provided to the anesthetist during crises, supervising the nurses' roles and support, equipment, and many other factors. The captain of the ship will eventually have to shoulder not only his or her own responsibility but also that of every other caregiver involved in the operating room.

I believe that going beyond the legal focus of operating rooms can legitimize the romantic notion of the captain of the ship. The health-care environment is becoming increasingly complex, with physicians undertaking more leadership roles. Most surgeons are not prepared to take on these roles despite emerging evidence that effective clinical leadership yields superior clinical outcomes for both patients and health-care organizations.

The surgeons of the future must be institutional leaders. They will have to lead formal debates and discussions with all stakeholders to influence and impact policies at the macro level and the institutional level. Some of the issues that need addressing are fair allocation of resources, transparency, good clinical governance, quality and patient safety, audits and accountability, and structured training programs well integrated into care delivery.

The doctrine of the captain of the ship has been present for as long as ships have been sailing. The only difference is that in those days, ships were made of wood, and people were made of steel. Today, the ships are made of steel, and the people are made of glass. If you are to really assume the role of captain of the ship, you must develop the character and substance to honor that role. Surgeons must have the qualities and attributes required to be true leaders in order to face the humongous challenges in the discipline of surgery today.

Finale

Practicing in surgery has always been a struggle in trying to adjust one's sails to achieve one's objectives. The difficulty is that you have no control over the wind. It is therefore incumbent on us to ensure that the younger generations are adequately primed in their training by teaching them what we were not taught but have learned ourselves. This is an effort to better prepare them and make them into well-rounded professionals. In the end, you should ask how training has impacted your own environment. Were you able to make any meager difference in your setting? Are the trainees of today better off? Do they feel professionally and ethically competent? Are the practices in surgical discipline better today?

Times have changed, values have changed, and people have changed and become more savvy and egoistical. Unfortunately, this is a global phenomenon. It suggests a wider and deeper problem. It reflects widespread societal apathy, malaise, and changing values. Edmund Pellegrino sensed this much earlier and said, "The physician today is an employee with divided loyalties, whose self-interest is pitted against the patient to curb costs and to make profits. Their professional worth is measured in productivity. They are not held to moral standards higher than those of the general society in which they live."[34] This sums up the fundamental shift in our professional attitudes. If you act like a service

---

34   Edmund Daniel Pellegrino, "Medical Professionalism: Can It, Should It Survive?" *The Journal of American Board of Family Practice* 13, no. 2 (2000): 147–149.

worker, why would you expect to be treated as a professional? This may have been a typical reflection of a practice model and societal practices in the United States. But it is no different in many other parts of the world. The comodification of medicine and deteriorating professionalism are also common in other countries around the world.

To play the devil's advocate, one may ask, are we expecting too much from our professionals? Are we not a part of the same society, with all its hypocrisy and prevailing scruples? Why do we expect physicians to be judged by higher moral standards?

Physicians must stand tall above everything around them. We need to be judged differently than any other profession. We are in the business of helping suffering humans, and this is not a small matter. Professionally and ethically, whatever we do or don't do impacts the lives of our patients and their families. We cannot allow surgery to slide down into a free-for-all situation on one pretext or the other. If you decide to join this profession, then you must commit yourself to higher values, expectations, and scrutiny.

We are the gatekeepers for people aspiring to enter this profession. It is therefore our responsibility to select and choose well from desirous candidates. High school and university grades have become the primary criteria (in some places, the only criteria) for entry into the profession. Grades are important, but they are only snapshots of the individuals we are recruiting. Cohorts come from diverse backgrounds and have variable degrees of moral development. We need to give equal—if not more— importance to somehow ascertaining the character of the individual. Does he or she have the required, essential humane attributes? This is a tough question, but it should be a necessary consideration for selection. This process is like selecting precious stones and then cutting them into gems; some will be more valuable than others, but they will still all be gems.

However, we must not be impatient about the issue of impact, for we are steering a ship here and not spinning a racing car around. It will take some time before the scene changes on the horizon, provided we continue to keep steering in the right direction. There is another pessimistic view emerging due to prevailing societal degradation: the idea that bioethics does not matter. Unfortunately, if we accept these thoughts, we are doomed as professionals and as a profession. After all, we have not stopped imparting to our children the basic human ethical values and tenets of living a decent, ethical life. Why would we stop doing so in a profession that actually deals with human lives?

Finally, it is worth reflecting on the fact that societies and values unfortunately change, and every new era seems to be worse than the one before. Elders have always lamented about the present, reminiscing about the good old days. This cycle will continue generation after generation. These days of our younger generation will become their good old days. It is our collective responsibility to ensure that we make the present of our young generation as memorable and educational as possible. The memory of it should be enough for them to impact newer generations and cherish their education in their old age.

Fortunately, there are many idealistic, dedicated, and great human beings still present among us who continue to shoulder this responsibility. They continue to impact future souls to carry the baton forward into the next generation. The world is a better place due to the existence of such people. They continue to do things to make a little difference in the world around them. They do this single-mindedly and irrespective of the outcomes, rewards, or recognition. These are the saviors and the rays of hope in every generation. We need to clone them in droves in our profession and in every generation. They are vital for the survival and future of our discipline of surgery, of our profession, and of humanity.

Afterword

Being a Surgeon conveys important messages. Through vivid examples, it tells us that medical professionalism isn't just a concept but is an actual, lived experience for the surgeon, who is called upon to respond appropriately to ethical challenges and make the right decisions in everyday surgical practice. Practice requires competence. This competence can be taught and learned. Dr. Raja provides sound advice to trainees and to trainers based on his personal experiences.

The book has an understandable slant toward practice conditions in resource-poor settings—the author's turf. This brings up two intriguing thoughts. Do the principles of medical professionalism that have been developed in the industrialized world apply just as well in resource-constraint situations? Are the environmental factors that influence professionalism any different?

Health care in resource-poor settings is by no means uniform. Broadly, there is the public sector, which supposedly caters to the majority of the population, and the private sector, which only the privileged and a small but rising middle class can afford. So how do the principles of medical professionalism apply in these sectors?

As far as upholding the primacy of patient welfare is concerned, there is probably greater accountability in the private sector, because private providers and the generally more informed citizenry patronizing these institutions tend to hold physicians more accountable. By contrast, the role of the national regulatory authority that ought to hold physicians accountable wherever they are is insignificant.

Autonomy, which is a relatively new concept even in the West, is generally on shakier ground in the developing world. Notwithstanding the higher educational level of patients in the private sector, there is a distinct Eastern culture called into play. Withholding information from the patient is customary, and there is undue deference to the doctor's decision and the decision of family members.

Distributive justice does not cross the divide between the two sectors—it isn't meant to! Each sector has its form of inequities. In private institutions, the quality of care is often directly proportional to the ability to pay. The state puts far more money into curative care than into prevention; all and sundry cannot access curative care, and the resources at its disposal are generally inferior to those in the private sector.

Market forces, technology, and health-care delivery systems conspire to undermine medical professionalism. Although this happens in the developed world, too, the scale of the undermining is much more in developing countries; and the environmental factors, which differ in some ways, are less amenable to fixing.

The way out of the logjam for resource-poor environments is medical education. However, education needs the solid support of institutional, national, and global policies to promote environments that are conducive to a high level of professionalism in practice. This brings us full circle back to the first point that the book makes about medical professionalism being an eminently teachable and learnable competence.

This book reflects Dr. Raja's angst in the face of the many challenges and diverse infringements of professional conduct he encounters in the discipline of surgery in whose service he has devoted an entire career. I hope his sincerity will rub off on readers as they embark on their own missions of furthering professional conduct.

Dr. Mushtaq Ahmed, MBBS FRCS
Professor of Surgery and Associate Dean of Medical Education
Aga Khan University, East Africa
December 3, 2016